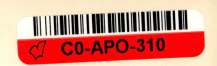

# A Synopsis of
# MEDICINE
## in
# DENTISTRY

# A Synopsis of
# MEDICINE
# in
# DENTISTRY

LAWRENCE COHEN, Ph.D., M.D., B.Ch.D., F.D.S.R.C.S. (Eng.)

*Professor and Head, Department of Oral Diagnosis, University of Illinois, Chicago; Director of Dental Education, Illinois Masonic Medical Center, Chicago; Consultant in Oral Diagnosis, Veterans Administration West Side Hospital, Chicago, Ill.; Consultant in Medicine, School of Dental Medicine, Southern Illinois University, Edwardsville, Ill.*

Lea & Febiger    •    *Philadelphia*    •    1972

*To my Wife, Gloria, and Sons, Alan, Martin and David*

*for their patience and forbearance during*

*the writing of this book*

# PREFACE

Before a dental student commences the study of Oral Pathology it is customary for him to take a course in General Pathology in order that he may apply the principles of pathology to oral conditions. Similarly, before he begins lectures in Oral Medicine he should have completed a course in the principles of Internal Medicine. He will then have acquired a broad background of the clinical manifestations of disease and treatment. The purpose of this book is to give the student this knowledge and to increase his professional stature and ability as a dentist.

There is some confusion within the dental profession concerning the terms 'oral diagnosis' and 'oral medicine.' Diagnosis implies the art of recognition of a disease but once the condition is recognized it is also necessary to treat it. Oral medicine includes both the diagnosis and the non-surgical treatment of oral disease. It is for this reason that the term 'oral medicine' is preferable to 'oral diagnosis.'

Within the past decade there has been a vast increase in medical knowledge with the result that it is becoming increasingly difficult for dentists to keep abreast of the latest developments. There are few dentists in practice who do not have patients with medical problems. My experience on both sides of the Atlantic has shown the need for a textbook which sets out the principles of internal medicine and discusses medical problems and their influence on dental treatment. In the text an attempt has been made to emphasize physiologic and pharmacologic principles and their relationship to the clinical manifestations of disease and treatment.

A section of commonly prescribed drugs together with some of their side effects has been included.   In addition, a chapter on the medical aspects of head injuries has been incorporated into the text.

Throughout the text an attempt has been made to place more emphasis on the common conditions encountered in practice.   However, the study of rare diseases has often provided much useful information of normal physiology.   When it was considered important to understand the underlying defects in less common conditions such as the hemoglobinopathies these have been explained in more detail.

I wish to thank Dr. Lee A. Malmed, Dr. Lawrence M. Solomon and Dr. Gerald A. Williams for contributing photographs, and Mrs. Maria E. Ikenberg of the Photographic Department of the Illinois Eye and Ear Infirmary for her expert assistance with the illustrations.   My thanks are also due to Miss Patricia Hall of Medical Illustrations, University of Illinois, for the excellent drawings.

This textbook is meant to be used in conjunction with ward rounds and with many excellent medical teaching films which are currently available. There is, however, no substitute for a patient.

LAWRENCE COHEN

# CONTENTS

## CHAPTER 1

# INFECTIOUS DISEASES

Infectious diseases may be classified according to the etiologic agent: bacterial, viral, spirochetal and fungal. Some of the infectious diseases are discussed in other sections of this book: for example, the common cold, influenza and tuberculosis are reviewed under *Respiratory Diseases*.

Various terms will be used in the discussion of infectious diseases, a few of which follow. The incubation period, for example, is the time which elapses between the invasion of the tissues by the infecting organism and the onset of the clinical symptoms.

During the course of some of these infections a rash appears on the skin (exanthem) and in some of them an eruption appears on the mucous membranes (enanthem). In describing a skin rash the expressions below are used:

*Erythema.* A diffuse reddening of the skin.

*Punctate erythema.* Small points of redness.

*Macule.* A circumscribed discoloration of the skin which is not raised above the surface of the surrounding skin.

*Papule.* A small raised area which can be felt with the fingers.

*Vesicle.* A small blister occurring on the skin or mucous membranes.

*Bulla.* A large blister occurring on the skin or mucous membranes.

*Pustule.* A small elevation of the skin containing pus.

## BACTERIAL INFECTIONS

### Streptococcal Infections

Infections with Group A β-hemolytic streptococci include streptococcal tonsillitis and scarlet fever. The incubation period is two to four days.

1

## STREPTOCOCCAL TONSILLITIS

Streptococcal tonsillitis differs from scarlet fever only in that the latter is due to infection with an erythrogenic strain of the organism in a nonimmune person. The erythrogenic toxin is responsible for the punctate erythematous rash and the characteristic enanthem.

## SCARLET FEVER

The typical enanthem consists of markedly red and edematous tonsils and stippling of the palate. The tongue is also coated with white fur through which the enlarged papillae stand out—the so-called "strawberry tongue." When the white fur peels off, the tongue has a red color—the "raspberry tongue." The cheeks are flushed and there is circumoral pallor. The exanthem follows within 24 to 36 hours and consists of a fine punctate erythema.

LABORATORY DIAGNOSIS. A sterile swab is rubbed over each tonsillar area and the posterior pharynx. To avoid contaminating the swab, the tongue or lips are not touched. The organism is grown on blood agar, and typically clear hemolysis occurs around the colonies after 18 to 24 hours' incubation.

TREATMENT. Penicillin is the drug of choice and is usually given for 10 days to prevent acute glomerulonephritis. In penicillin-sensitive patients erythromycin is given.

### Diphtheria

Diphtheria is caused by *Corynebacterium diphtheriae* and has an incubation period of one to three days. The organism has no invasive power and the threat to life results entirely from the effect of the toxin on the heart, nerves and adrenals.

CLINICAL FEATURES. The local lesion of diphtheria on the mucosa of the pharynx, larynx or trachea is characterized by the formation of a false membrane. The organism causes surface necrosis of the mucosa which combines with the fibrinous exudate to form a "membrane" which is strongly adherent to squamous epithelium but is loosely attached to ciliated epithelium. The exudate on the tonsil may resemble a streptococcal or Vincent's infection. Most diphtheritic lesions have a characteristically offensive pungent odor. There is congestion and edema of the surrounding structures. Periadenitis involving the connective tissue around the lymph nodes gives rise to the classical "bull-neck" of diphtheria.

Diphtheria toxin may affect the myocardium causing toxic myocarditis between the eighth and tenth day; the first signs are tachycardia and an irregular pulse. The motor nerves may be affected producing palatal, pharyngeal, laryngeal and ocular paralysis. Kidney involvement may cause albuminuria and in severe cases renal failure. Acute adrenal insufficiency results in fall of the blood pressure, vomiting and hemorrhagic rashes (Waterhouse-Friderichsen syndrome).

TREATMENT. Diphtheria antitoxin is given as early in the disease as possible.

PROPHYLAXIS. Active immunization will prevent diphtheria and is normally effected in children by three injections of alum precipitated toxoid at one-month intervals. It is usual to give a combined triple vaccine (DPT) against diphtheria, pertussis (whooping cough) and tetanus.

The Schick test is used to detect whether a person has immunity against diphtheria. The test is performed by injecting into the skin of the forearm 0.1 ml. of diluted highly purified diphtheria toxin. The development of a variable area of redness at the site of inoculation over a period of 72 to 120 hours signifies a positive reaction and indicates that the patient is susceptible to the disease. A negative Schick test signifies that the subject is unlikely to contract clinical diphtheria.

## Whooping Cough (Pertussis)

Whooping cough is caused by *Bordetella pertussis* and *Bordetella parapertussis* and has an incubation period of one to two weeks. It is one of the most serious of the acute specific fevers of childhood.

CLINICAL FEATURES. After what appears to be a common cold, a harsh cough develops and becomes progressively more severe. Paroxysms of coughing (during which a series of explosive coughs occurs) are followed by a prolonged inspiration through a partly closed glottis. This gives rise to a characteristic "whoop." Following a series of paroxysms the child often vomits or coughs up thick mucus. During a spasm of coughing the child may abrade the lingual frenum against the lower incisors thus causing a frenal ulcer, or he may rupture a blood vessel in the conjunctiva giving rise to a subconjunctival hemorrhage. In the respiratory tract bronchopneumonia and areas of collapse of the lung (atelectasis) may occur which in later life may result in bronchiectasis.

LABORATORY DIAGNOSIS. There is a lymphocytosis of 15,000 to 45,000. The typical colonies can be cultured on Bordet-Gengou medium containing penicillin held in front of the patient's mouth during a paroxysm of coughing.

TREATMENT. Tetracycline, chloramphenicol, streptomycin and erythromycin have been used. The child should be fed immediately after he has vomited to prevent weight loss.

PROPHYLAXIS. Active immunization with triple (DPT) vaccine will prevent an attack.

## VIRAL INFECTIONS

### Measles (Rubeola, Morbilli)

Measles is caused by a paramyxovirus and is highly contagious. The disease has a tendency to occur in epidemics every second year in the late winter and early spring.

CLINICAL FEATURES. After an incubation period of 10 to 14 days the disease begins with fever, sneezing, running nose, red eyes and a cough. In over 90 percent of the patients pinhead-sized, grayish spots on an erythematous background appear on the buccal mucous membrane in the region of the molar teeth. Known as Koplik's spots, these areas constitute the enanthem; their number varies from only a few to many such spots.

On the third day the skin rash appears behind the ears at first, and then it spreads to the face and trunk. Usually a mild general lymphadenopathy may be noted. The rash from the onset is maculopapular, with round or oval lesions which tend to become confluent and give the characteristic blotchy appearance of measles. As the rash fades it leaves a brownish staining of the skin associated with desquamation and the temperature falls to normal. Complications of measles are most often due to secondary bacterial infection and include otitis media and bronchopneumonia.

TREATMENT. There is no specific treatment for measles. The child is kept in bed, and any complications are treated with the appropriate antibiotic.

PROPHYLAXIS. Active immunization is obtained by the injection of measles vaccine at 12 months of age or older. Passive immunization is usually conferred by giving gamma globulin within the first few days after exposure has occurred.

## Rubella (German Measles)

Rubella occurs mainly in children and adolescents. The incubation period is 12 to 23 days.

CLINICAL FEATURES. German measles begins with fever, catarrh and conjunctivitis and is followed within 24 hours by a generalized, pinkish macular rash. The latter appears first on the forehead and behind the ears and then spreads over the rest of the body. Characteristically the posterior cervical lymph nodes are enlarged. A few petechiae may occur on the soft palate. The disease is usually mild and self-limiting.

Twenty percent of the children born to mothers who have had rubella in the first trimester of pregnancy have congenital defects such as cataract, congenital heart disease, deafness and mental retardation.

DIAGNOSIS. Leukopenia is frequently found in rubella. Isolation of the virus from throat washings in the first 24 hours can be carried out.

TREATMENT. Treatment is symptomatic.

PROPHYLAXIS. Living vaccines containing virus attenuated by serial passage in tissue culture are injected subcutaneously and will protect against rubella. In the last few years a single subcutaneous injection of a combined vaccine containing live rubella, measles and mumps viruses has been used to protect against all three diseases.

## Herpesvirus Infections

The herpesviruses include the causative agents of herpes simplex and the varicella-zoster virus, the causative agent of chickenpox and herpes zoster.

# HERPES SIMPLEX

The herpes simplex virus is distributed widely throughout the community. In many cases infection with the virus takes place during the first few months of life while the baby is protected by maternal antibodies and produces a subclinical infection with no clinical disease. After the loss of maternal antibodies the child becomes susceptible to the clinical disease on his first encounter with the virus.

## Primary Herpetic Infections

These may involve the skin, mucous membranes, conjunctivae or the central nervous system and are usually severe. Eczema herpeticum (Kaposi's varicelliform eruption) is a primary manifestation of herpesvirus infection of the skin of a patient with eczema.

## Acute Herpetic Stomatitis

Acute herpetic stomatitis usually occurs in children between six months and five years of age but may also be seen in adolescents and adults. Crops of vesicles occur throughout the oral cavity including the gingiva. These vesicles soon rupture, leaving ulcers which become secondarily infected. Typically the child is febrile and cannot eat or drink because of the sore mouth. Healing of the ulcers occurs within 10 to 14 days.

LABORATORY DIAGNOSIS. Provided the lesions have been present for less than two to three days, the typical multinucleated giant cells and giant nuclei are seen; intranuclear inclusions are rare.

TREATMENT. Local applications of 5-iodo-2′-deoxyuridine (IDU) have been used in the treatment of herpetic infections, as IDU interferes with the metabolism of the virus. It has not been as successful as was anticipated. Antibiotics are given to control secondary infection. A soft diet with plenty of liquids is of value. Fruit juices, because of their acidity, cause pain in the early stages of the disease and should be avoided.

## Recurrent Herpetic Infections

It is believed that following the primary infection the herpesvirus lies dormant in the tissues and is activated from time to time by fevers, exposure to sunlight or menstruation. The recurrent lesions tend to occur around mucocutaneous junctions and are thus found around the lips and nose (herpes labialis or herpes febrilis). The patient experiences a burning sensation in the area, and at the site of irritation a number of thin-walled vesicles appear. These soon rupture and a scab forms which heals without scarring within the next seven days. The lesions have a marked tendency to reappear at the same site. Recurrent herpetic lesions may also occur intraorally.

TREATMENT. There is no specific treatment. An antibiotic cream such as neomycin cream can be applied to reduce secondary infection and to promote healing.

## VARICELLA (CHICKENPOX)

Chickenpox is an acute infectious disease caused by a virus which is identical with the virus of herpes zoster. The incubation period is 13 to 17 days. The onset is sudden with fever and the rash appearing together. In children the systemic symptoms are usually mild and complications are rare, but in adults the disease may be more severe.

CLINICAL FEATURES. The eruption begins as small, discrete, irritant red papules which in a few hours turn into thin-walled vesicles containing clear fluid. The vesicles become pustular within 48 hours. During the next two days they dry up to form scabs which soon fall off. The fever usually subsides within two to three days of the onset.

Characteristically the vesicles appear first on the back and chest and then on the lower trunk where they are more numerous than on the face and extremities. The lesions occur in crops so that papules, vesicles and crusts are all present at the same time. This distinguishes chickenpox from smallpox where the lesions are all at the same stage. The oral mucous membrane is frequently affected, and the lesions are rather similar to those of herpes simplex.

LABORATORY DIAGNOSIS. Multinucleated giant cells and inclusion bodies similar to herpes simplex and herpes zoster are found on exfoliative cytologic examination.

TREATMENT. Calamine lotion is used to prevent itching. A phenolic mouthwash is soothing when oral lesions are present.

## HERPES ZOSTER (SHINGLES)

In herpes zoster the virus affects a posterior root ganglion, the gasserian ganglion or the geniculate ganglion. The incubation period is short. Within three to seven days after exposure to the virus, the patient experiences a continuous burning pain in the area of the skin supplied by the sensory nerves involved. Two or three days later crops of vesicles appear, and the surrounding skin is inflamed and edematous. The majority of cases occurs in the thoracic area. The rash is almost invariably unilateral.

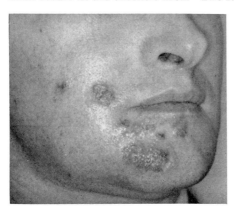

**Figure 1.1.** Herpes zoster. Before the lesions appeared, the patient experienced pain for 24 hours at the site of the skin eruption. The lesions which are now crusted are confined to the mental nerve distribution. Male, aged 29 years.

## Herpes Zoster of the Gasserian Ganglion

The maxillary division of the fifth nerve and the mental nerve may be involved by herpes zoster. In both cases, intraoral vesicles are present in the distribution of the involved nerve (Figure 1.1).

## Ophthalmic and Geniculate Herpes (p. 172)

TREATMENT. There is no specific treatment. Analgesics are used to control the pain. Antibiotic creams may be used to prevent secondary infection.

## Smallpox (Variola)

Smallpox is caused by the variola virus, one of the poxviruses. The poxviruses that affect man are the variola, vaccinia, cowpox and molluscum contagiosum viruses.

The variola virus is carried from patient to patient in infected skin secretions or contaminated dust. When inhaled, it reaches the upper respiratory tract where it multiplies in the lymphatic tissues. The incubation period is seven to thirteen days.

CLINICAL FEATURES. Smallpox is ushered in by a high fever (102°–103°) associated with severe toxemia. On the third or fourth day numerous lesions appear on the oral and pharyngeal mucosa, face and hands and then spread to the trunk and lower limbs. The trunk is involved to a variable extent, but the axillae and groins are spared. This distinguishes the rash from chickenpox which is maximal over the trunk and the lesions of which come out in crops.

The eruption in smallpox begins with macules which change into papules, then into vesicles and finally pustules over a period of four to seven days. In the late vesicular stage of smallpox depressed, "umbilicated" vesicles are seen. The pustulation and the fever which occur during the latter part of the eruptive stage are due to secondary bacterial infection and can be controlled to some extent by the use of antibiotics.

Variola minor (alastrim) is a milder form of smallpox and the mortality rate is much lower than in classical smallpox (variola major).

LABORATORY DIAGNOSIS. Serologic tests are employed in the diagnosis of smallpox but are not as reliable as growing the virus on the chorioallantoic membrane of a chick embryo where the typical pocks appear within seventy-two hours.

TREATMENT. Treatment is largely symptomatic. Antibiotics are given to control secondary infection.

PROPHYLAXIS. Vaccination with the vaccinia virus will prevent smallpox and is employed in the prevention of epidemics. Methisazone, an antiviral compound, has also been used in the prophylaxis of smallpox.

2

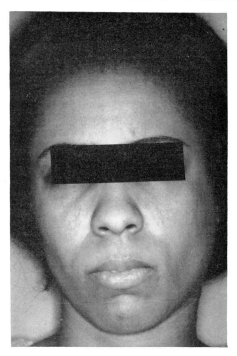

**Figure 1.2.** Unilateral mumps. The patient complained of pain and swelling in the left parotid region for the previous 24 hours. Clear saliva was expressed from the left parotid duct thus excluding a bacterial infection of the gland. The S antibody was raised, establishing a diagnosis of mumps. The right parotid gland did not enlarge Female, aged 29 years.

## Mumps (Epidemic Parotitis)

Mumps is caused by the mumps virus, a member of the myxovirus group and is spread by inhalation of droplets. The incubation period is eighteen to twenty-one days. Children and adolescents are most commonly affected.

CLINICAL FEATURES. There is painful swelling of one parotid gland, and within twenty-four hours the other gland enlarges. Mumps is most often bilateral but may be unilateral (Figure 1.2). The submandibular and sublingual salivary glands are occasionally involved. An early sign of mumps is redness of the parotid papilla, but no discharge can be expressed from the parotid duct. The incidence of involvement of testes, pancreas, breast and ovaries increases with age. The fever usually subsides in three to five days and the patient makes a complete recovery in the next seven to ten days.

LABORATORY DIAGNOSIS. Complement fixing antibodies are produced and are of two types: the S antibody, which appears rapidly during the first week of illness, reaches a peak, then gradually wanes, and the V antibody, which is slower to form but persists longer. By means of antibody tests it is possible to make a firm diagnosis of mumps. As parotitis may rarely be caused by other viral infections such as Coxsackie A and lymphocytic choriomeningitis, antibody tests are of importance in establishing the causative virus.

TREATMENT. Treatment is symptomatic. Analgesics may be prescribed to control the pain.

PROPHYLAXIS. A single injection of a live attenuated mumps virus vaccine gives protection in more than 95 percent of susceptible people.

## Herpangina

Herpangina is caused by the Coxsackie A viruses.

CLINICAL FEATURES. The illness begins suddenly with anorexia, fever up to 104° F, and occasionally vomiting. The pharynx is hyperemic and there are minute vesicles occurring mainly on the anterior pillars of the fauces but extending onto the soft palate, uvula, tonsils, tongue, buccal mucosa and occasionally the gingivae. The vesicles soon rupture and leave shallow ulcers one to two mm. in diameter, each with a grayish base and an erythematous margin. Healing usually occurs within seven days.

Herpangina should be differentiated from hand, foot and mouth disease which is also associated with the Coxsackie A virus and in which a vesicular eruption involves the hands, feet and mouth.

LABORATORY DIAGNOSIS. The causative virus may be isolated from swabs taken from throat lesions or from fecal specimens.

TREATMENT. Treatment is entirely symptomatic.

## Infectious Mononucleosis

Infectious mononucleosis, an infectious febrile disease, is probably caused by a herpes-like virus and most commonly affects young adults. It has a short course and is characterized by lymphadenopathy, sore throat and liver damage.

CLINICAL FEATURES. After an incubation period of four to twenty days the disease is ushered in with headaches, sore throat and increasing fever (103° to 105° F) and toxemic symptoms. The sore throat varies in intensity from a mild inflammatory reaction to a severe anginose exudative pharyngitis which resembles diphtheria. Oral ulceration may occur and resemble that of agranulocytosis or acute leukemia. A cluster of small hemorrhages at the junction of the hard and soft palates may be observed. There is usually discrete and firm enlargement of the cervical, axillary and inguinal lymph nodes. The spleen may be slightly enlarged. In about five percent of cases a maculopapular rash appears during the first ten days of the illness.

LABORATORY DIAGNOSIS. The total leukocyte count is usually 10,000 to 20,000 per cu. mm. Characteristically there is an increase of mononuclear cells of various types and these may comprise 80 to 90 percent of the total leukocyte count. Also present are many large atypical lymphocytes which have a deep blue staining foamy cytoplasm and oval- or kidney-shaped nuclei with coarsely stranded and fenestrated chromatin, the "glandular fever cells."

Serologic testing may be done for a heterophil antibody which is present in the serum of many infectious mononucleosis patients and causes the agglutination of sheep's red cells. This antibody is distinctive in that it can be absorbed by ox erythrocytes but not by a suspension of guinea pig kidney tissue.

TREATMENT. Treatment is almost entirely symptomatic; bed rest is recommended.

### Viral Hepatitis

There are two forms of viral hepatitis, infectious hepatitis and serum hepatitis.

## INFECTIOUS HEPATITIS

Occurring mainly in children and adolescents, infectious hepatitis is spread by fecal contamination. After an incubation period of fifteen to forty days, the disease manifests with fever, anorexia and malaise followed by nausea, vomiting and diarrhea. During this stage the liver is tender and may be slightly enlarged. In many cases the cervical lymph nodes are enlarged. Within five to seven days jaundice appears and deepens. Recovery is slow over a period of four to six weeks during which time the patient is frequently depressed and lethargic.

LABORATORY DIAGNOSIS. Serum transaminase (glutamic-oxaloacetic and glutamic-pyruvic) levels are markedly raised early in the disease. The abnormal liver function tests return to normal during convalescence.

## SERUM HEPATITIS

The incubation period of serum hepatitis is 40 to 160 days. The virus is most frequently transmitted in blood transfusions and in injections with inadequately sterilized needles and syringes. The symptoms resemble those of infectious hepatitis.

LABORATORY DIAGNOSIS. Recently a virus-like antigen (Australian antigen or serum hepatitis antigen) has been identified in the blood during the incubation period and early clinical course of post-transfusion hepatitis. The antigen usually disappears with clinical recovery.

In serum hepatitis the liver function tests are abnormal as in infectious hepatitis.

TREATMENT is bed rest and supportive diet in both forms of viral hepatitis.

PROPHYLAXIS. Gamma globlulin protects against or modifies infectious hepatitis in exposed subjects. There is conflicting evidence concerning the value of gamma globulin in the prophylaxis of serum hepatitis. To reduce the risk of post-transfusion hepatitis blood donors should be carefully selected.

## SPIROCHETAL INFECTIONS
### Syphilis (Lues)

The causative organism of syphilis is *Treponema pallidum*, and the disease is most frequently acquired through sexual intercourse. Shortly after infection immunity begins to develop, and two distinct antibodies appear in the serum at this time. One of these is syphilitic reagin which is closely associated with the plasma gamma globulins and provides the basis for the flocculation and complement fixation tests for syphilis. The other antibody is the treponemal antibody.

CLINICAL FEATURES

*Primary syphilis.* Ten to ninety days (average twenty-one days) following infection a chancre develops at the site of treponemal invasion. Chancres most frequently occur on the genitals but may occur on the fingers and in the oral cavity. They are usually single but multiple lesions can occur. The lesion, which may vary in size from a few millimeters to two centimeters in diameter, is usually an eroded papule which is firm on palpation. The surface may be crusted or ulcerated. Typically the chancre is painless unless it is secondarily infected. The draining lymph nodes are usually enlarged, firm and painless (Figure 1.3). Within one to five weeks of its appearance the chancre heals spontaneously. The serologic tests for syphilis are usually nonreactive when the chancre first appears but become reactive during the following one to four weeks.

*Secondary syphilis.* About six weeks after the chancre first appears the secondary stage of syphilis is ushered in by a sore throat, generalized lymph node enlargement, skin rashes and mucous patches. The latter are grayish, translucent lesions occurring in the mouth and other mucous membranes and are highly infective. Large hypertrophic papules, con-

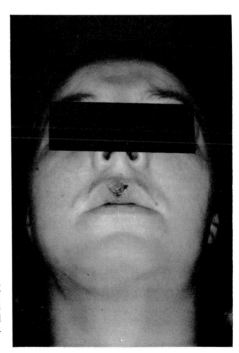

**Figure 1.3.** Primary chancre of lip. The patient complained of an ulcer of the upper lip which had been present for two weeks. Note the bilateral submandibular lymphadenopathy. Female, aged 32 years.

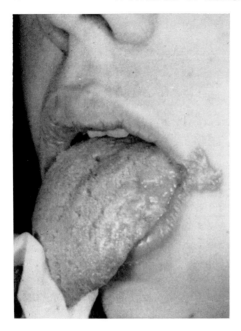

**Figure 1.4.** Secondary syphilis. Split papules representing the secondary stage of syphilis are present at the commissures of the mouth. The lesions are more proliferative than angular cheilitis resulting from an infection with *Staphylococcus aureus* from which they must be differentiated. Female, aged 22 years.

dylomata lata, may occur in the anogenital region and in skin folds. Split papules at the angles of the mouth resemble angular cheilitis (Figure 1.4). (The serologic tests during this stage are positive. Within two to six weeks the secondary lesions heal but the serologic tests remain reactive.)

*Latent syphilis.* Following the secondary stage the patient enters the latent period. This may last a lifetime or be followed from a few years to twenty years or more by lesions of tertiary syphilis. No lesions are present in latent syphilis, and the only sign of infection is a reactive serologic test.

*Tertiary syphilis.* Approximately one third of the people with untreated syphilis will develop late destructive lesions of syphilis which include gummas, cardiovascular complications and central nervous system involvement.

A gumma may occur singly or be multiple. Gummas may occur anywhere but are most commonly found in the mucocutaneous tissues, liver, bones and testes. They are probably the result of hypersensitivity reaction to the treponemal infection and result in a rubbery, grayish white, necrosis of the tissue (Figure 1.5).

In cardiovascular syphilis, luetic involvement of the aorta results in weakening and scarring of the media with consequent dilatation of this vessel (aneurysm formation). Widening of the aortic valve ring results in aortic regurgitation and stenosis of the mouths of the coronary vessels causes angina pectoris. Cardiovascular complications account for 80 percent of the deaths.

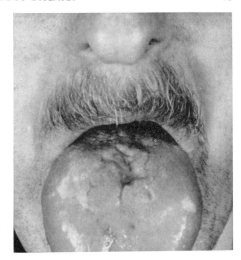

**Figure 1.5.** Gumma of tongue. Note the midline, punched-out lesion of the tongue which had been present for one month and was slightly painful. In addition there are areas of leukoplakia on the dorsum of the tongue. Male, aged 65 years.

For a discussion of central nervous system involvement in tertiary syphilis, see page 174.

*Congenital syphilis.* Infection of the fetus occurs at about the fifth month of intrauterine life. Syphilis may result in spontaneous abortion or produce well-recognized stigmata. Within the first few weeks of life the child may develop a skin rash mainly around the mouth and anus and desquamation of the palms and soles. The mucous membrane of the nose and pharynx are frequently involved and the child has a heavy mucoid discharge known as snuffles. A hemorrhagic nasal discharge in the newborn period is characteristic of syphilis. Following healing of the oral lesions radiating scars or rhagades may occur around the mouth.

A generalized syphilitic osteochondritis and periochondritis affects all bones of the skeletal system, particularly the nose and lower limbs. Destruction of the vomer leads to a saddle nose. New bone growth on the anterior surface of the tibia produces anterior bowing or a saber tibia.

If congenital syphilis is untreated in about 60 percent of the patients the disease is latent with no manifestations other than a reactive serologic test for syphilis. In the remainder, interstitial keratitis (a ground glass appearance of the cornea), Hutchinson incisors which are typically screwdriver-shaped, Moon's molars (maldevelopment of the cusps of the first molars) and eighth nerve deafness occur.

*Oral aspects.* The chancre may involve the lips, tongue, gingivae or tonsils. Mucous patches occur in the oral cavity during the secondary stage. A gumma of the tongue results in a rubbery swelling usually in the midline which breaks down leaving a punched-out ulcer. In the hard palate, a gumma occurs typically in the midline and leads to perforation. Hutchinson incisors and Moon's molars occur in congenital syphilis.

LABORATORY DIAGNOSIS. If the surface of the chancre is cleaned and the serum expressed from it examined with darkfield microscopy, *Treponema pallidum* can be identified by its morphologic characteristics and its typical motion. Care must be exercised in interpreting darkfield examination of material from the oral cavity as some saprophytic spirochetes have similar characteristics to *T. pallidum*.

All diagnostic tests for syphilis depend on the reaction of antibody with antigen. The tests may be divided into nontreponemal or reagin tests where the antigen is an extract from normal tissue or other sources and the treponemal tests which employ treponemes or treponemal extracts to detect antibody. The term "serologic test" usually refers to nontreponemal antigen tests. The Venereal Disease Research Laboratory (VDRL) slide test is one which is employed routinely in diagnosis. It should be noted that false positive reactions occur in a number of unrelated clinical states such as measles, chickenpox, infectious mononucleosis, the other spirochetal infections and any febrile illness. The Treponema Pallidum Immobilization test of Nelson will be positive in other treponematoses.

Following treatment of tertiary syphilis there is little or no change in the serologic tests. In neurosyphilis a reactive VDRL test is obtained on the spinal fluid.

TREATMENT. Penicillin is the drug of choice. In patients who are sensitive to penicillin, erythromycin or the tetracyclines are used.

PROPHYLAXIS. Patients who have been exposed to infectious syphilis should receive treatment. If a pregnant woman is found to have a positive serologic test she should be treated immediately to prevent infection of the fetus.

## FUNGAL INFECTIONS

### Candidiasis

Several types of the genus *Candida* infect man, but *Candida albicans* is probably the most common. *Candida* tends to affect patients who are malnourished or have an underlying disease such as diabetes or a malignancy. It may occur in pregnancy or in patients receiving corticosteroid or antibiotic therapy. Candidal infections of the skin, lungs and kidneys have been reported but are rare.

ORAL ASPECTS. Acute candidiasis (thrush) and chronic forms of candidiasis such as angular cheilitis, denture stomatitis and candidal leukoplakia occur.

TREATMENT. Nystatin tablets 500,000 units are sucked q.i.d. or nystatin suspension can be applied q.i.d. to the lesions. Treatment may extend over four to six weeks or longer.

### Actinomycosis

Infection with the microorganism *Actinomyces israeli* may occur in the cervicofacial, thoracic and ileocecal regions. Actinomycetes are normally present in the mouth. The disease is characterized by the formation of suppurating lesions in the tissues and chronic sinuses. In early cases the typical sulfur granules may be expressed from the skin lesions.

TREATMENT. Penicillin is the drug of choice. Tetracyclines can be used in penicillin-sensitive individuals.

## Histoplasmosis

Infection with the causative organism, *Histoplasma capsulatum,* in most patients results in a relatively asymptomatic pulmonary infection. In a proportion of cases lesions of the oral mucosa occur. These consist of chronic ulcers and granulomas. Histologic examination of biopsy specimens reveals large numbers of histiocytes containing the spores of *Histoplasma.*

TREATMENT. Intravenous amphotericin B is effective.

## GENERAL REFERENCES

Ramsay, A. M. and Edmond, R. T. D.: *Infectious Diseases,* London, Heinemann, 1967.
Slobody, L. B. and Wasserman, E.: *Survey of Clinical Pediatrics,* 5th ed., New York, McGraw-Hill, 1968, pp. 203–263.
*Syphilis, a Synopsis,* Public Health Service Publication, No. 1660, January 1968.

## CHAPTER 2

# ALLERGY AND IMMUNE REACTIONS

Allergy may be defined as an altered capacity of the body to react to various antigens with which it comes into contact. An antigen is a substance that induces the formation of antibodies or of sensitized cells. Ordinarily, antibodies to constituents of the host's own tissues are not produced.

Some simple organic compounds, while in themselves nonantigenic, may combine with larger molecules to produce an antigen. These simple compounds are called haptens, and the larger molecules—generally a protein or polypeptide—are known as the carriers.

Those antigens which are responsible for clinical allergic manifestations are usually referred to as allergens. The latter may be inhaled, ingested, injected or absorbed through the intact skin. Drugs containing foreign protein, such as liver extract and horse serum, may themselves induce an allergic reaction, whereas drugs such as penicillin are haptens and become antigenic when combined with host protein.

## Antibody Formation

Antibody formation occurs in the reticuloendothelial system of the spleen, lymph nodes, bone marrow and other organs containing lymphoid tissue, with the exception of the thymus. It is now believed that the thymus functions by providing cells which populate the antibody-forming tissues where they divide into clones of cells capable of responding to antigen.

The plasma cell is considered to be involved in the synthesis of antibody. There is evidence that cells of the lymphocytic series, which are of importance in delayed hypersensitivity, also play a role in antibody formation, It has also been suggested that the small lymphocytes may provide "immunologic memory."

## HYPERSENSITIVITY

The local or systemic reactions which affect the host animal on exposure to antigens are referred to as hypersensitivity. Two types of hypersensitivity are recognized: immediate and delayed. In immediate hypersensitivity, the antigen reacts with the antibody, either by entering the circulation or by being fixed to certain tissues thus causing the formation or release of chemical substances which produce the reactions. As immediate hypersensitivity is caused by circulating antibodies, the reaction can be produced in normal recipients by injection of the serum of an affected individual followed by challenge with the antigen. These antibodies can generally be localized to one of the three immunoglobulin fractions of the serum (IgG, IgA, IgM). In delayed hypersensitivity, there are immunologic responses involving reaction of antigen with specifically sensitized cells. Hence, this type of hypersensitivity is passively transferrable with sensitized cells but not with serum or antibody.

### Immediate Hypersensitivity

Two types of immediate hypersensitivity will be discussed and these are anaphylaxis and serum sickness.

### ANAPHYLAXIS

Occasionally patients who are given an injection of serum or a drug, e.g. penicillin, may collapse and die within minutes. Asthmatic wheezing, cyanosis and severe pruritus often occur at the onset of the reaction. This is known as anaphylaxis.

TREATMENT consists of the intravenous or intracardiac administration of epinephrine, external cardiac massage and the administration of oxygen.

### SERUM SICKNESS

Seven to ten days after an injection of a foreign serum or protein, the patient may manifest a reaction that is characterized by fever, skin eruptions of which urticaria is the most common, lymphadenopathy and joint pains. Although the manifestations of serum sickness appear some days after administration of antigen, they are mediated by antibody and, hence, the disease is a form of immediate hypersensitivity.

TREATMENT. Urticaria usually responds to small doses of epinephrine and can be controlled with ephedrine and antihistamines. Joint pains respond to aspirin. Steroids are also of value and are given for five to seven days.

## Delayed Hypersensitivity

In delayed hypersensitivity, or cellular immunity, exposure to the antigen results in an inflammatory reaction which develops maximally over the injection site 24 to 48 hours after injection. A typical example of delayed hypersensitivity is the tuberculin reaction.

Allergic contact dermatitis is a form of delayed hypersensitivity. The drug which is applied to the skin acts as a hapten and combines with dermal protein to produce an antigen. Patch testing with the specific compound is used to confirm the diagnosis.

Rejection of homografts is a form of delayed hypersensitivity.

## Drug Allergy

Allergy to drugs may be the result of immediate or delayed hypersensitivity. One form of immediate hypersensitivity which has already been discussed is anaphylactic shock resulting from the injection of penicillin.

Without exception, any drug systemically administered is capable of causing a skin eruption or an oral eruption.

*Aspirin* can cause urticaria.

*Antibiotics.* In general, candidal overgrowth occurs in the oral, genital and anal orifices. Also with penicillin, urticaria and erythema multiform-like eruptions occur.

*Barbiturates.* Urticarial, erythematous, bullous, purpuric and fixed drug eruptions have been reported.

## ALLERGY TO DENTURE BASE MATERIAL

Allergy to denture base material is very rare. Redness under dentures is more likely to be caused by ill-fitting dentures and candidal infections.

## Allergic Rhinitis (p. 25)

## DERMATOLOGIC ALLERGY

Under this heading are included urticaria, angioneurotic edema, contact dermatitis, stomatitis venenata, atopic eczema and drug eruptions. The term "eczema" is used to describe a group of eruptions in which erythema, vesicle formation and crusting are the principal features. The term "dermatitis" indicates an inflammatory condition of the skin. Frequently the terms "eczema" and "dermatitis" are used synonymously and interchangeably.

## Urticaria

Urticaria is an eruption of the skin characterized by transitory, sharply demarcated, elevated, flat-topped wheals usually accompanied by erythema and itching. The urticarial wheal is the result of edema of the dermis, arises as the result of histamine release and is inhibited by antihistamines.

Urticaria may be due to a variety of causes among which is an allergy to food or drugs. Stress and emotional factors may also play a part.

TREATMENT. Antihistamines are of value.

### Angioneurotic Edema (Angioedema)

Transitory, localized, painless swellings of the subcutaneous tissue or submucosa of various types characterize angioneurotic edema. It occurs in two forms, a rare *hereditary* form and the more common *sporadic* type. The latter is essentially a giant form of urticaria and is due to the same causes as urticaria. Occasional cases of angioedema may be caused by aspirin.

CLINICAL FEATURES. The lesion is most often single but may be multiple. It consists of a tense, nonpitting, rounded swelling a few centimeters or more in diameter. The edema is localized but lacks the sharply defined, raised border of urticaria. The overlying skin is usually normal in color and temperature but may be slightly reddened. There is no pain but there may be slight itching. The chief sensation is one of distention. The face, hands, feet and genitalia are the skin areas most often affected (Figure 2.1).

TREATMENT is with antihistamines.

### Contact Dermatitis (Dermatitis Venenata)

This is a very common inflammation of the skin caused by the exposure of the skin either to primary irritant substances such as soaps or to allergenic substances such as poison ivy. Erythema, vesicles and bullae are found and the lesions may become secondarily infected (Figure 2.2).

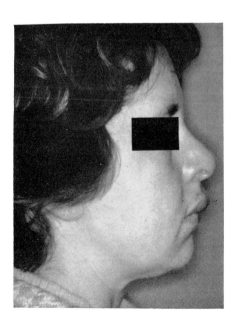

**Figure 2.1.** Angioneurotic edema. The upper lip had swelled on a number of occasions. There is now some permanent enlargement. Female, aged 37 years.

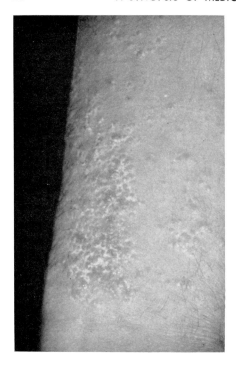

**Figure 2.2.** Contact dermatitis. Numerous vesicles are present on the flexor surface of the forearm of this patient resulting from contact with poison ivy. Male, aged 26 years. (*Courtesy of Dr. Lawrence M. Solomon*)

TREATMENT is corticosteroid creams or systemic corticosteroids in severe cases.

### Stomatitis Venenata

Contact allergy can occur on the lips and in the oral cavity from contact with lipstick, mouthwashes and toothpaste. When the lips are involved, the condition is termed cheilitis venenata.

TREATMENT. On the lips corticosteroid creams are used. Patients with severe oral lesions are given systemic corticosteroids.

### Atopic Eczema (Atopic Dermatitis)

Atopic eczema is a rather common, markedly pruritic, chronic skin condition. Frequently the patient has a family history of asthma, hay fever and atopic eczema.

CLINICAL FEATURES. There are two clinical forms, infantile and adult. In the infantile form, blisters, oozing and crusting with excoriation occur; the lesions are found on the face, scalp, arms and legs or may be generalized. In the adult form, marked dryness of the skin with thickening (lichenification), excoriation and even scarring occurs. The lesions are found on the cubital and popliteal fossae, on the dorsum of the hands and feet or may be generalized. The infantile form usually becomes milder or even disappears after the age of three or four years. At the age of puberty and the late teens, flare-ups or new outbreaks can occur (Figure 2.3).

TREATMENT. Local treatment with corticosteroid and other creams.

### Drug Eruptions

As stated previously any drug when systemically administered may cause a skin eruption (dermatitis medicamentosa) or oral lesions (stomatitis medicamentosa).

TREATMENT is with local or systemic corticosteroids.

## AUTOIMMUNITY

Autoimmunity is the ability of the body to react immunologically to its own normal constituents resulting in the production of antibody and/or sensitized lymphoid cells.

In man, autoimmunity is associated with two main groups of diseases. The first group is the *organ specific immune diseases* in which the body reacts to constituents normally present in, and peculiar to, the affected organ. Among the diseases in this group are Hashimoto's thyroiditis (p. 132), and primary adrenocortical atrophy (idiopathic Addison's disease, p. 138). In the second group of diseases, the autoimmune responses are directed against a normal body constituent found in many or all organs and tissues. The *connective tissue diseases* ("collagen diseases") are included in this group, and the lesions observed affect the cells and ground substance of

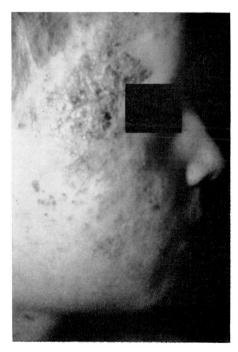

**Figure 2.3.** Atopic eczema. Note the crusted lesions on the face of this six-year-old boy. (*Courtesy of Dr. Lawrence M. Solomon*)

the connective tissue.  Members of the group include rheumatoid arthritis (p. 154), systemic lupus erythematosus, progressive systemic sclerosis (diffuse scleroderma), rheumatic fever (p. 48), dermatomyositis and polyarteritis nodosa (periarteritis nodosa).  Sjögren's syndrome has been associated with each of the connective tissue diseases (p. 111).

## Lupus Erythematosus

The two principal varieties of lupus erythematosus are the chronic discoid form and the systemic form.  It has been shown that patients with systemic lupus erythematosus produce various antinuclear antibodies which can be detected by special tests.  The "LE phenomenon" consists of the demonstration in the bone marrow or peripheral blood of clusters of polymorphs around lysed nuclear material; the LE cell is a polymorph which has engulfed a mass of homogeneous nucleoprotein.

### CHRONIC DISCOID LUPUS ERYTHEMATOSUS

In this condition chronic erythematous areas appear over the cheeks and nose producing a butterfly distribution.  Over the affected areas are found thin scales associated with plugging of the pilosebaceous follicles.  The affected skin is scarred.  The oral mucosa may be involved producing areas of erosion with a white margin due to hyperkeratosis (Figure 2.4).

TREATMENT.  Chloroquine, an antimalarial, is taken orally.

### SYSTEMIC LUPUS ERYTHEMATOSUS

Systemic lupus erythematosus occurs more frequently in young females.  It is associated with a generalized macular rash with a high fever.  Loss of hair, albuminuria, arthritis, leukopenia and reversal of the albumin-globulin ratio of the blood occur.  There is generalized lymphadenopathy and splenomegaly, and erosions of the buccal mucosa may also be present.  The disease is frequently fatal.

TREATMENT.  Large doses of corticosteroids are given.

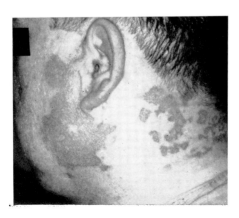

Figure 2.4.  Chronic discoid lupus erythematosus.  The affected skin is atrophic and thin scales are present on the surface of the lesions.  Male, aged 30 years.  (*Courtesy of Dr. Lawrence M. Solomon*)

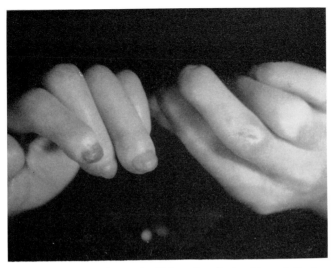

**Figure 2.5.** The skin of the fingers is thickened and atrophic and the hands in this advanced case are clawed (sclerodactyly). Female, aged 61 years.

## Progressive Systemic Sclerosis (Diffuse Scleroderma)

In this disease there is a diffuse sclerosis of the skin, subcutaneous tissue and other organs. In some patients localized skin lesions (morphea) occur. In others the scalp is involved, and sclerosis and scarring produce a picture which resembles a saber wound (coup de sabre).

CLINICAL FEATURES. Females are affected more commonly than males and the disease tends to develop during middle age. Following fever and joint pains the skin of the face, the upper part of the trunk or the limbs becomes pink, smooth and waxy. Later, it becomes white and adheres to the underlying tissue. The face, if affected, is immobile and the patient may have difficulty in opening his mouth. In about 90 percent of cases the hands are affected and become clawlike (sclerodactyly) (Figure 2.5). Subcutaneous calcification may occur. When the esophagus is affected dysphagia results. Intestinal involvement may result in the malabsorption syndrome.

TREATMENT. Systemic corticosteroids are of value.

### GENERAL REFERENCES

Glynn, L. E. and Holborow, E. J.: *Autoimmunity and Disease*, Philadelphia, Davis, 1965.
Lewis, G. M. and Wheeler, Jr., C. E.: *Practical Dermatology*, 3rd ed., Philadelphia, W. B. Saunders, 1967.

### SUGGESTED READING

Bickley, C. H.: Immunity and oral disease: a synopsis of the science of immunity. JADA, *79*, 368, 1969.

## CHAPTER 3

# DISEASES OF THE RESPIRATORY SYSTEM

It is conventional to divide the respiratory tract into two parts, upper and lower. The upper respiratory tract is comprised of the nasal cavity, nasopharynx and larynx. The trachea, bronchi and lungs constitute the lower respiratory tract. Each lobe of the lung is subdivided into a number of broncho-pulmonary segments each of which is supplied by a segmental bronchus.

## DISEASES OF THE UPPER RESPIRATORY TRACT

### Common Cold

The common cold is an acute, highly communicable infection of the upper respiratory tract. The most important causative agents are the rhinoviruses. Infection is spread from one patient to another by inhalation of droplets and the incubation period is from one to two days. Colds are more frequent in the fall and winter.

CLINICAL FEATURES. The patient complains of irritation in the throat soon to be followed by a nasal congestion and then a watery nasal discharge accompanied by sneezing. The eyes are reddened and frequently the speech has a nasal quality. Secondary bacterial invaders give rise to a purulent nasal discharge and occasionally such complications as tracheo-bronchitis, ear infections, sinusitis, laryngitis and pneumonia occur.

TREATMENT. There is no specific treatment. Rest, analgesics and de-congestant nose drops are employed.

## Influenza

Influenza is an acute respiratory disease caused by the influenza virus of which there are three distinct antigenic types, designated A, B and C. Infection with one type confers no immunity against infection from the other two. The disease is spread by inhalation of infective droplets and the incubation period is usually from 18 to 36 hours. Influenza A viruses are the cause of major epidemics.

CLINICAL FEATURES. The onset is sudden, the most common initial symptom being severe frontal headache. The patient feels ill, and chilliness and fever with pains in the muscles are associated with the disease. The temperature rises quickly to between 100° and 103° F and there is usually an unproductive cough. The face is flushed and the skin hot and dry; the patient sneezes, his eyes water, and his throat is red.

The chief complications of influenza are secondary infections of the middle ear, paranasal sinuses, bronchi and lungs.

TREATMENT. Bed rest and analgesics are employed. Secondary bacterial infections are treated with the appropriate antibiotics.

PROPHYLAXIS. Vaccines are now available which will protect the patient against an attack of influenza.

## Allergic Rhinitis

Allergic rhinitis may be seasonal or perennial. The seasonal type (hayfever or pollinosis) is usually caused by pollens from trees, grasses or flowers. It lasts several weeks, then disappears to return the following year. Perennial rhinitis is due to sensitivity to a variety of allergens, such as house dust, and may occur throughout the year. Large numbers of eosinophils are found in the nasal secretion.

CLINICAL FEATURES. The usual symptoms of allergic rhinitis are nasal obstruction, sneezing and a profuse watery nasal discharge. The allergic nose shows a a bluish-white appearance of the nasal mucosa.

TREATMENT. The best treatment for allergic rhinitis is to find the allergen and then eliminate it. This, however, is not always possible. A course of desensitization injections is often helpful in the seasonal type but not in the perennial type. Antihistamines are of value during an attack.

## Vasomotor (Nonallergic) Rhinitis

Some patients complain of chronic nasal obstruction or stuffiness which is not due to allergy; this condition is called vasomotor rhinitis. In some cases, this is the result of overuse of nasal drops which initially clear the nasal passages. Later, there is compensatory relaxation of the blood vessels of the turbinates and further stuffiness. One cause of nasal obstruction is deviation of the nasal septum and symptoms may disappear after surgery. Frequently patients with vasomotor rhinitis have underlying emotional problems which make treatment difficult.

## Acute Laryngitis

Acute laryngitis may occur during the course of the common cold or as an isolated infection.

CLINICAL FEATURES. The throat is sore and the voice is hoarse. Later, the patient may lose his voice altogether. Cough is usually present but is non-productive unless there is an associated tracheitis and bronchitis. Small children may have a brassy cough with associated swelling of the mucous membrane which can cause obstruction of the airway. The patient with acute laryngitis does not always have a raised temperature.

TREATMENT. Bed rest. Talking must be forbidden to rest the larynx. The patient should not smoke. Steam inhalations, hot gargles and drinks give relief. Cough is treated with a cough suppressant. Rarely, if obstruction is present, tracheostomy may be necessary.

## Chronic Laryngitis

Chronic laryngitis is liable to occur in those people such as singers and public speakers who constantly use their voices. Excessive use of tobacco and alcohol are often predisposing factors. Chronic sinusitis may also make the patient susceptible to chronic laryngitis.

CLINICAL FEATURES. Hoarseness is the chief symptom. Pain is absent or minimal. The patient usually coughs frequently. Examination of the larynx shows the vocal cords to be thickened and red.

It is essential to examine the larynx in patients with persistent hoarseness which has been present for more than three weeks to exclude papilloma, carcinoma, cord paralysis or, more rarely, tuberculosis or syphilis.

TREATMENT. The voice should be rested. Smoking and alcohol should be forbidden. Steam inhalations are of value. Biopsy of the cords may be necessary to distinguish between laryngitis and neoplasm.

# DISEASES OF THE LOWER RESPIRATORY TRACT

## Examination of the Chest

Examination of the chest is customarily carried out in the following order—inspection, palpation, percussion and auscultation.

## INSPECTION

The chest is inspected to see if any abnormality is present. In emphysema, the anteroposterior diameter is increased and the chest expansion is reduced. It is important to observe any difference in movement between the two sides of the chest.

CLUBBING OF THE FINGERS. The fingers should be inspected for the presence of clubbing, the earliest change of which is a filling in of the angle between the skin at the base of the nail and the nail itself. Later the fingers become club-shaped. Clubbing is observed in cyanotic congenital heart disease, bacterial endocarditis, carcinoma of the bronchus and in chronic suppurative conditions such as bronchiectasis and lung abscess. In some patients, clubbing is familial and there is no underlying disease (see Figure 4.1).

## PALPATION

The trachea is felt to determine whether it lies in the midline in the suprasternal notch. In fibrosis of the lung, the trachea is pulled towards the affected side. A large collection of fluid in one side of the chest will push the mediastinum and trachea to the opposite side.

## PERCUSSION

The chest is percussed to learn whether any change in the percussion note has taken place. Impaired resonance is found over collapsed, consolidated or fibrosed lung while hyperresonance is found over a pneumothorax (air in the pleural cavity).

## AUSCULTATION

The quality of the breath sounds is ascertained with the stethoscope. *Vesicular breath sounds* are the sounds heard over normal functioning lung tissue. *Bronchial breath sounds* are the sounds heard normally over the bronchi. In bronchial breathing, expiration is louder, longer and of higher pitch than inspiration, in contrast to vesicular breathing in which inspiration is longer. Bronchial breath sounds are heard over areas of consolidation of the lung. *Rales* are interrupted crackling sounds produced by air passing through fluid in the respiratory tract. A *rhonchus* is a continuous, somewhat musical noise produced by air passing through a narrowed bronchus.

## Bronchitis

Bronchitis is inflammation of the mucous membrane lining the bronchi and may be either acute or chronic.

## ACUTE BRONCHITIS

Acute bronchitis usually follows acute tracheitis. When both occur simultaneously, the condition is termed acute tracheobronchitis. Acute bronchitis and tracheobronchitis usually complicate colds, influenza, measles and whooping cough.

CLINICAL FEATURES. Acute tracheitis causes soreness behind the sternum and a dry, painful cough. When the infection involves the bronchi, the patient wheezes and has difficulty in breathing. As secondary bacterial infection occurs, a thick, purulent sputum is produced. The condition produces a variable degree of malaise being more serious in young children and older, debilitated patients.

TREATMENT. In mild cases bed rest, steam inhalations and a cough suppressant will suffice. In young children and the elderly, particularly in the presence of some underlying disease, antibiotics are indicated.

## CHRONIC BRONCHITIS

Chronic bronchitis is a disease which affects mainly males between the ages of 30 and 60. It is related to heavy smoking, air pollution and long-term inhalation of dust. In the early stages, the bronchial mucous glands and the goblet cells of the bronchial epithelium undergo hypertrophy. Later, ulceration of the bronchial mucosa is found and secondary infection tends to occur. Purulent sputum may be produced from which *Haemophilus influenzae* or pneumococci are frequently cultured.

CLINICAL FEATURES. The patient frequently complains of an early morning cough associated with the production of a non-infected sputum which he ascribes to smoking. Over the years, the quantity of the sputum and the duration of the cough increase until the patient is rarely free of symptoms. A winter cold may result in an exacerbation of the disease with the production of purulent sputum occasionally tinged with blood. The patient experiences increasing dyspnea which at first is due to secretions or bronchospasm and later to the development of emphysema. Some patients become so breathless on slight exertion that they are unable to work. Auscultation reveals generalized rhonchi due to narrowing of the bronchi. A radiograph of the chest in chronic bronchitis may show no abnormality unless emphysema is present.

TREATMENT. The patient should stop smoking and, if possible, move to a warm, dry climate. He should stay at home when he has a cold or in foggy weather. During attacks, the oral administration of bronchodilators, expectorant mixtures and antibiotic drugs is of value and may shorten the period of disability.

## ACUTE BRONCHIOLITIS

This is an acute inflammation of the bronchioles occurring usually in infants and small children. It produces obstruction leading to difficulty in breathing (dyspnea) and occasionally may be fatal.

TREATMENT is bed rest, oxygen and the appropriate antibiotic.

### Emphysema

Emphysema is a disease of the lungs which is characterized by pathologic enlargement of the distal air spaces due to dilatation or destruction of their walls. These changes result in a loss of elasticity of the lungs and produce obstruction to the air flow which manifests clinically as dyspnea. Many of the etiologic factors of chronic bronchitis apply equally well to patients with emphysema.

CLINICAL FEATURES. Typically, the patient gives a history of chronic bronchitis and his major complaint is persistent breathlessness. In well-established cases the anteroposterior diameter of the chest increases.

Chest expansion, however, is diminished. The accessory muscles of respiration, particularly the sternocleidomastoids, are frequently employed during inspiration and the patient breathes through pursed lips. Percussion over the heart and liver shows diminished dullness in these areas because of the air-filled lung overlying these organs. The breath sounds are faint. In advanced cases with associated chronic bronchitis, normal alveolar gas exchange is impaired and the patient is cyanosed. The hypoxemia leads to pulmonary vasoconstriction and an increase in arterial resistance. The work of the right side of the heart is increased and cor pulmonale ensues (right ventricular hypertrophy).

TREATMENT. The treatment of bronchial infection and bronchospasm is the same as for chronic bronchitis. In addition patients are taught breathing exercises to improve the respiratory exchange.

## Bronchiectasis

Bronchiectasis is a condition which is characterized by dilatation of the bronchi. It usually results from prolonged bronchial obstruction and infection. The latter causes disruption of smooth muscle and elastic tissue and, in addition, the ciliated epithelium is destroyed and is replaced by cuboidal epithelium. The other factor necessary in the genesis of bronchiectasis is an increase in outward traction of the surrounding lung tissue.

Some cases may be of congenital origin as bronchiectasis occurs in about 20 percent of parents with dextrocardia (Kartagener's syndrome). These patients usually have chronic sinusitis.

In the child, bronchiectasis may complicate whooping cough and measles or aspiration of a foreign body. Carcinoma of the bronchus may, by obstructing the bronchus, cause atelectasis (collapse) and infection and produce bronchiectasis in the adult.

CLINICAL FEATURES. Cough and purulent sputum are the classic symptoms. Hemoptysis (the expectoration of blood, by coughing, from the respiratory tract) may also occur. Blood-streaked sputum is the most common form of hemoptysis but occasionally severe bleeding occurs. Recurrent acute exacerbations of respiratory infection are usual, often initiated by upper respiratory infection such as the common cold. Clubbing of the fingers may also be present. In the chest crepitations are heard over the bronchiectatic area. These are produced by the opening of alveoli filled with exudate or by air bubbling through mucus in bronchi of various sizes. In addition there may be signs of collapse, fibrosis or pneumonia.

The dilatation of the bronchi can be demonstrated by bronchograms (radiographs taken after the bronchi have been filled with radiopaque fluid). TREATMENT. Medical treatment consists of chemotherapy and postural drainage. The latter consists of tipping the patient to drain the bronchiectatic area into the bronchi and trachea so that he can expectorate the secretions. Surgical treatment is resection of the affected area.

## Asthma

Asthma is characterized by attacks of expiratory dyspnea and wheezing due to bronchial spasm and accumulation of secretions in the bronchi. About one-third of patients with asthma have a family history of an allergic disorder such as hay fever, asthma or urticaria. When seasonal, the disease is most likely to be caused by allergy to inhaled pollen. Nonseasonal asthma may be the result of allergy to dust, feathers, animal fur, foods or drugs. Aspirin may induce an attack of asthma in sensitive individuals, as may infection and emotional disturbances. Skin testing is helpful in finding the allergen.

Asthma starting later in life is often found not to be allergic in origin.

CLINICAL FEATURES. During an attack, the patient has difficulty in breathing associated with wheezing. At first there is a dry unproductive cough but later in the attack the sputum becomes more liquid and easier to expectorate. A severe attack lasting more than one day is known as status asthmaticus. Auscultation of the chest shows widespread rhonchi, particularly on expiration. After an attack, the patient's lung function returns to normal.

TREATMENT. Bronchodilators may be taken orally or by inhalation of an aerosol preparation. Subcutaneous injection of 0.5 ml. of 1:1000 epinephrine can also be employed. Morphine should never be given during an attack. In status asthmaticus, corticosteroids may be lifesaving.

Between attacks the patient should avoid contact with the allergen. In some cases the patient can be desensitized for the particular allergen which provokes an attack.

## Carcinoma of the Bronchus

This disease is one of the most common causes of death in the United States and Europe. The increased incidence of bronchogenic carcinoma in cigarette smokers has been substantiated. Air pollution is also a factor, the incidence of the disease being higher in industrial than in rural areas. In addition, there is a higher incidence in miners who are exposed to dusts from nickel, chromium and radioactive ores. In the majority of patients, the tumors arise within an inch or two of the bifurcation of the trachea. In the remainder, the lesions are peripheral. The most common histologic types are the squamous cell and the anaplastic.

CLINICAL FEATURES. Because of the association with cigarette smoking, patients with bronchial carcinoma often have chronic bronchitis and as a result may have had morning cough for many years. However, a recent increase in severity of cough should arouse suspicion. The expectoration of blood-tinged sputum may occur and in some cases frank hemorrhage results from the ulceration of a blood vessel.

Narrowing of the bronchus by the tumor will result in collapse of the lung segment supplied by the affected bronchus and the patient may complain of breathlessness. Secretions in the affected bronchus are retained and may become infected. As a result, a segmental pneumonia may occur and a lung abscess may form in the affected area.

Some patients complain of pain in the chest resulting from invasion of the pleura or chest wall by carcinoma.

In addition to the respiratory symptoms the patient may complain of tiredness, anorexia and loss of weight.

Tumors in the region of the apex of the lung may involve the cervical sympathetic and give rise to Horner's syndrome (p. 161). These apical tumors may also involve the brachial plexus and cause pain in the arm and shoulder. The supraclavicular lymph nodes may be involved as well.

Carcinomatous infiltration of the mediastinal lymph nodes and pleura may give rise to a pleural effusion which is often blood-stained. Bronchial carcinoma frequently metastasizes to the liver, lymph nodes, brain and bones. A metastasis in a bone may weaken it to such an extent that it fractures (pathologic fracture) with minimal trauma. Although metastases to the jaws have been reported from carcinoma of bronchus, they are rare.

Clubbing of the fingers occurs frequently in carcinoma of the bronchus. Hypertrophic pulmonary osteoarthropathy may also occur and includes periosteal new bone formation, mainly in the long bones, and swelling and pain in the joints. A radiograph will show typical subperiosteal new bone formation at the distal ends of the long bones.

DIAGNOSIS. A radiograph of the chest and bronchoscopy with biopsy of the lesion will confirm the diagnosis (Figure 3.1).

TREATMENT. Surgical removal of the affected lobe or lung offers the best chance of cure. Radiotherapy and cytotoxic drugs are also employed in patients unsuitable for surgery.

## Metastatic Tumors of the Lung

The lung is a common site for metastatic tumors, which are usually spread by the bloodstream. Sarcomas, such as those of bone, frequently

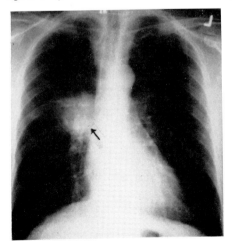

Figure 3.1. A bronchogenic carcinoma of the right upper lobe with enlarged adjacent hilar lymph nodes form a confluent large mass on the right (arrow). Male, aged 56 years. (*Courtesy of Dr. Lee A. Malmed*)

produce metastases in the lungs, as do also the renal tumors, hypernephroma (adenocarcinoma) and embryonal adenosarcoma (Wilms' tumor). Usually multiple discrete nodular tumor masses are seen on the chest radiograph.

TREATMENT. If there is a discrete lesion it may be possible to resect the affected portion of the lung. Usually the treatment is palliative because of the advanced nature of the disease.

## The Pneumonias

Pneumonia is an inflammation of the lung which results in consolidation of lung tissue. The pneumonias may be classified on the basis of the infecting organism and on the anatomic distribution. The term pneumonitis is used synonymously with pneumonia. There are two main types of pneumonia—lobar pneumonia and bronchopneumonia.

## LOBAR PNEUMONIA

In lobar pneumonia one or more lobes of the lung undergoes consolidation. The pneumococcus is the most common causative organism.

CLINICAL FEATURES. Pneumococcal lobar pneumonia may occur at any age. The disease is usually ushered in by a rigor and the temperature rises rapidly. The patient's face is flushed and there may be herpes labialis. Over the consolidated lobe, the pleura becomes inflamed and this is known as pleurisy. The latter causes pain on respiration and, as a result, the breathing becomes rapid and shallow. The patient usually has a painful cough and his sputum may be blood-tinged.

During the early stages of the disease, examination of the chest may reveal little except diminished movement on the affected side together with

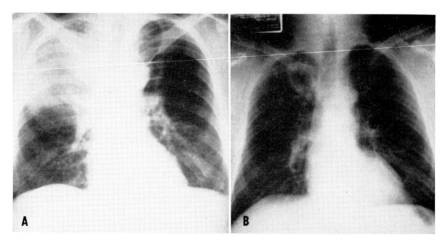

**Figure 3.2.** **A.** Lobar pneumonia, right upper lobe. Note the radiopacity caused by the inflammatory process. **B.** A follow-up film made approximately one month later shows almost complete resolution of the process. Male, aged 47 years. (*Courtesy of Dr. Lee A. Malmed*)

reduced breath sounds. Within 24 to 48 hours, the signs of lobar consolidation appear which may be confirmed by a radiograph of the chest (Figure 3.2) and which results in dullness on percussion and changes in the breath sounds. Polymorphonuclear leukocytosis is associated with lobar pneumonia.

TREATMENT. In the preantibiotic era in those patients who recovered, a crisis occurred and the temperature fell abruptly on about the seventh day. Today antibiotic treatment modifies the course of the disease and the patient responds within 48 hours of commencing therapy.

COMPLICATIONS. Pneumococcal pneumonia rarely leaves any damage to the lungs. Slow resolution may be due to underlying conditions such as carcinoma or bronchiectasis. Effusions into the pleural cavity may occur and, on occasion, these may become purulent resulting in empyema. Lobar pneumonia due to such organisms as the tubercle bacillus, Friedländer's bacillus (*Klebsiella pneumoniae*) or the staphylococcus may progress to lung abscess and subsequent fibrosis.

## BRONCHOPNEUMONIA (LOBULAR PNEUMONIA)

In bronchopneumonia, the consolidation of lung tissue is of a lobular type, occurs in both lungs and tends to be patchy and irregular in distribution. Bronchopneumonia may be caused by bacteria, fungi, rickettsiae and viruses and tends to occur more often in the two extremes of life. In the young, it often complicates acute infectious diseases such as measles, whooping cough and scarlet fever. In the elderly, bronchopneumonia is often a terminal disease. It may follow aspiration of foreign bodies or infected material during anesthesia and unconsciousness.

CLINICAL FEATURES. The onset of the disease may vary from a minimal systemic upset to a fulminating infection. Pleurisy may occur and give rise to pain on respiration. The sputum is purulent and may be blood-stained. The temperature is raised and fluctuates, but rarely reaches normal and this is described as a remittent fever.

Examination of the chest may often reveal little more than bilateral patches of impaired resonance, reduced breath sounds and rales. A radiograph of the chest will confirm the presence of patchy consolidation (Figure 3.3).

TREATMENT. In the bacterial pneumonias, the diagnosis is confirmed by sputum culture and antibiotic sensitivities of the organism. Before the bacteriologic reports are available, it is usual to commence treatment with intramuscular penicillin providing the patient is not allergic to the drug. If the infecting organism is found to be insensitive to penicillin, the antibiotic can be changed. Pleuritic pain can be treated with injections of meperidine or morphine. Cough is relieved by codeine.

In pneumonias due to inhalation of infected material, aspiration of the tracheobronchial tree is necessary together with postural drainage and the administration of antibiotics.

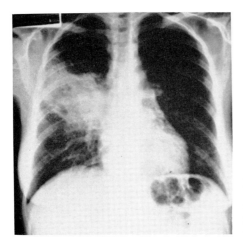

**Figure 3.3.** Bronchopneumonia. Infiltrates are seen involving the right lower lobe in both its superior and basilar segments as well as in the right upper lobe. Note the breast shadows in this 36-year old female. (*Courtesy of Dr. Lee A. Malmed*)

## Lung Abscess

The commonest cause of lung abscess is the aspiration of infected material from the respiratory passages. About 80 percent of patients with an aspiration abscess have poor oral hygiene. Aspiration of blood clot or a tooth fragment may occur as a complication of tonsillectomy and following tooth extraction particularly under general anesthesia. Bronchial obstruction secondary to carcinoma of the bronchus with associated infection may give rise to lung abscess.

CLINICAL FEATURES. The patient presents with fever, malaise and night sweats followed by pain in the chest and a dry cough. After some days, the abscess discharges into a bronchus and the patient coughs up large quantities of foul-smelling sputum, sometimes mixed with blood. The abscess may rupture into the pleural cavity resulting in empyema. Clubbing of the fingers develops in a proportion of cases.

There is usually dullness on percussion over the affected area associated with impaired breath sounds. A radiograph of the chest will confirm the diagnosis.

LABORATORY DIAGNOSIS. Laboratory findings show a polymorphonuclear leukocytosis. Culture of the sputum will reveal the causative organism and enable the antibiotic sensitivities to be determined.

TREATMENT. Penicillin is given initially until the results of the sputum examination are available. Postural drainage will assist in the withdrawal of the purulent material. Some patients will require surgery to eradicate the infection.

## Tuberculosis

Tuberculosis is a disease caused by *Mycobacterium tuberculosis*. The two most important strains in human disease are the human and bovine, of which the human bacillus is the most common cause of tuberculosis in Europe and the United States.

Infection with the tubercle bacillus in a host who has never been previously exposed to the organism is called primary tuberculosis. When the patient has been previously infected and reinfection occurs, this form of the disease is called postprimary tuberculosis. Two theories exist concerning the pathogenesis of this form: reactivation of a previous focus of the disease may occur or reinfection may take place with organisms derived from outside the body.

MANTOUX TEST. An antigen prepared from dead tubercle bacilli (tuberculin) is injected intracutaneously. In those patients who have recently acquired tuberculosis and who have been previously infected with the disease, an antigen-antibody reaction occurs in the skin producing an area of redness and swelling. The test is read at 48 to 72 hours. Erythema is disregarded and the diameter of the induration is measured. Only reactions above 10 mm. are regarded as of tuberculous origin.

## PRIMARY TUBERCULOSIS

Tubercle bacilli form a focus of infection in the lung at their portal of entry. The lesion produced which is known as the *primary* or *Ghon focus* consists of typical tuberculous granulation tissue and this drains into the regional lymph nodes which become enlarged forming the *primary complex*. In the majority of patients, the primary complex heals with minimal symptoms. In a few instances there is rapid pathologic progression and tubercle bacilli may be spread via the bloodstream to other organs giving rise to miliary tuberculosis.

The Ghon focus is usually located just beneath the pleura and is found more frequently in the lower half of the lower lobe. Most of the lesions occur in the period from one to three years of age. The healed Ghon focus frequently calcifies.

In some instances, the primary focus may occur in the tonsil and the cervical lymph nodes become involved. The latter may caseate forming a tuberculous abscess but in most instances the nodes heal by fibrosis and calcification.

## POSTPRIMARY TUBERCULOSIS

Postprimary tuberculosis is often the result of reinfection in adult life. The infection is almost invariably pulmonary and usually occurs in the upper lobes. The early lesion is a small area of tuberculous lobar pneumonia which can be seen as a soft shadow on a radiograph (Figure 3.4). Tuberculous cavities result from softening and liquefaction of caseous lobar pneumonia. Spread of the disease may occur via the bronchi in addition to local extension. Subpleural lesions may invade the pleural cavity and cause pleurisy which may progress to an effusion or empyema. Aneurysmal

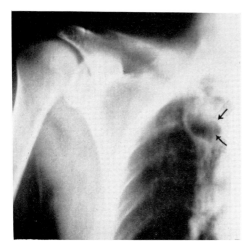

Figure 3.4. Postprimary tuberculo-sis. Tomograph. There is a cavity in the right apex of the lung surrounded by a thickened, irregular wall which represents a tuberculous abscess (arrows). A positive sputum for TB organisms was obtained. Male, aged 60 years. (*Courtesy of Dr. Lee A. Malmed*)

dilatation of a branch of the pulmonary artery in tuberculous cavities may occur and give rise to bleeding.

In some instances, pulmonary tuberculosis may progress throughout the lung causing gross fibrous contractions of the lung parenchyma. The result is dyspnea and cyanosis.

The expectoration of infected sputum may cause tuberculous tracheitis, laryngitis or tuberculous ulcers on the tongue. Tuberculous ulceration of the ileum may result from the swallowing of infected sputum.

CLINICAL FEATURES. Many patients are free of symptoms and their disease is detected on routine chest x ray. On occasion, hemoptysis may be the presenting symptom of an early lesion.

The classic symptoms of pulmonary tuberculosis are chronic ill health, cough, low grade fever, weight loss and night sweats.

Persistent rales may be heard over the affected area. If fibrosis occurs, there will be impairment to percussion and sometimes bronchial breathing.

Radiography is essential for diagnosis and for following the course of the disease.

TREATMENT. Bed rest. The antituberculous drugs—streptomycin, paraminosalicylic acid (PAS) and isoniazid—are administered.

## ORAL TUBERCULOSIS

Oral tuberculosis may be either primary or secondary to tuberculosis elsewhere in the body. In the primary form, which is very rare, a tuberculous lesion forms at the site of invasion of the oral tissues by the tubercle bacillus. The draining lymph nodes are enlarged. Tuberculous oral ulcers are most frequently secondary to tuberculosis of the lungs and are often painful. A definitive diagnosis may be established by histologic examination of a biopsy specimen. In addition a radiograph of the chest should be taken to exclude tuberculosis of the lungs.

## Sarcoidosis

The etiology of this disease is still unknown. Although it was thought that sarcoidosis was related to tuberculosis the histopathologic findings are different. In sarcoidosis, the epithelioid cell follicle often exhibits fibrinoid necrosis, but there is no true caseation as occurs in classic tuberculosis.

CLINICAL FEATURES. The disease tends to affect women between the ages of 18 and 25 slightly more than men of the same age group. Sarcoidosis appears in all socioeconomic groups of the population in contrast to tuberculosis which tends to occur in the economically depressed. The disease is often ushered in with polyarthritis or with reddish lumps (erythema nodosum) on the legs. Lung involvement is the most common and varying degrees of dyspnea and cough are noted. Almost any organ may be affected. Uveitis may occur and may produce visual impairment. Enlargement of the salivary glands occurs in less than 10 percent of cases and then usually regresses spontaneously. A syndrome of fever, uveitis, lacrimal and salivary gland enlargement is known as uveoparotid fever or Heerfordt's syndrome. Facial nerve palsy may also occur. Cysts form in the distal phalanges of the hands and feet in about 10 percent of cases. Skin lesions vary from small papules to extensive erythematous infiltrated and ulcerated lesions.

LABORATORY DIAGNOSIS. A radiograph of the chest may show involvement of the lungs and symmetric bilateral hilar adenopathy. The patient is hyposensitive to the tuberculin tests which distinguishes the disease from tuberculosis. In 50 to 80 percent of patients with sarcoidosis, the Kveim test (the intracutaneous injection of a heat-sterilized suspension of human sarcoid tissue) produces a nodular lesion. The nodule must be biopsied in four to six weeks to confirm the histologic picture of sarcoidosis. Patients with sarcoidosis may have hypercalcemia and hypercalciuria.

TREATMENT. Corticosteroids, chloroquine and butazolidin effectively suppress the granulomas of sarcoidosis.

## GENERAL REFERENCES

Crofton, J. and Douglas, A.: *Respiratory Diseases*, Philadelphia, F. A. Davis Company, 1969.

DeWeese, D. D. and Saunders, W. M.: *Textbook of Otolaryngology*, St. Louis, Mosby, 1960.

## CHAPTER 4

# DISEASES OF THE CARDIOVASCULAR SYSTEM

The heart and great vessels may be affected by congenital anomalies some of which may not manifest until adulthood. Disease of the cardiovascular system is one of the most common causes of death. Coronary artery disease and hypertension are found more frequently in the older age group and patients with these conditions are likely to be encountered among those receiving dental treatment.

## THE EXAMINATION OF THE CARDIOVASCULAR SYSTEM
### Cyanosis

One of the most important signs of cardiovascular disease is cyanosis which is the bluish color of the skin and mucous membranes caused by an excess of reduced hemoglobin. Five grams of reduced hemoglobin per 100 ml. are required to produce detectable cyanosis.

There are two types of cyanosis:

### PERIPHERAL CYANOSIS

This is best seen in the lips and extremities and is due to coldness of the part. It is never seen in the tongue or mouth.

### CENTRAL CYANOSIS

Central cyanosis affects the mouth and tongue as well as the extremities. It is due either to inadequate uptake of oxygen in the lungs secondary to pulmonary disease, or to a right-to-left cardiac shunt which results in deoxygenated blood bypassing the lungs and passing directly to the systemic circulation.

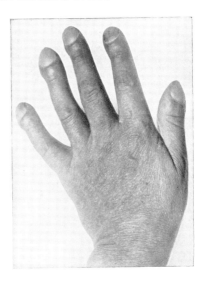

**Figure 4.1.** Clubbing of the fingers.

## Clubbing of the Fingers

Clubbing of the fingers is the term given to thickening around the nail-bed with filling in of the angle at the base of the nail; it can best be observed when the finger is viewed from the side. It is seen in congenital cyanotic heart disease, chronic chest infections such as lung abscess, bronchiectasis and empyema, carcinoma of the bronchus and cirrhosis of the liver (Figure 4.1).

## The Pulse

### RATE

The average rate of the pulse in normal adults is 60 to 80 per minute; in children, 90 to 140; in the aged, 70 to 80.

### TACHYCARDIA

Acceleration of the pulse, tachycardia, occurs during and after exercise, in emotional states and in fever. In anemia and after a severe hemorrhage, the pulse is markedly increased in rate. Hyperthyroidism will cause tachycardia which persists during sleep.

### BRADYCARDIA

Slowing of the pulse, bradycardia, occurs in myxedema, arteriosclerosis, jaundice and typhoid fever. Increased intracranial pressure will also cause a decrease in the pulse rate. In heart block, the pulse rate may be as low as 40.

In atrial fibrillation, the pulse is irregular in force and rhythm.

4

## Neck Veins

In heart failure and superior vena caval obstruction the neck veins are distended.

## Ankle Swelling

In heart failure abnormal retention of sodium in the tissue spaces takes place. The tissue fluid tends to settle under the influence of gravity into the most dependent parts of the body. Thus, the ambulant patient develops swelling of the feet and legs which is most marked in the evenings, whereas the patient confined to bed has a pad of edema overlying the sacrum. *Cardiac edema pits on pressure.*

The differential diagnosis of ankle swelling includes:

1. Renal disease
2. Deficient lymphatic drainage of the legs
3. Deep vein thrombosis of the legs or severe varicose veins
4. Cirrhosis of the liver
5. Ankle swelling in normal women after standing for much of the day and most marked in the premenstrual phase when sodium and water retention is greatest

## CONGENITAL CARDIOVASCULAR ANOMALIES

Congenital cardiovascular anomalies result from embryonic defects occurring during the period of development of the heart and great vessels. The most important of these anomalies may be classified as follows:

1. *Cyanotic Group*
   With right-to-left shunt:
   Tetralogy of Fallot
2. *Acyanotic Group*
   a. With left-to-right shunt:
   Persistent ductus arteriosus
   Atrial septal defect
   Ventricular septal defect
   b. Without shunt:
   Coarctation of the aorta
   Pulmonary stenosis
   Congenital aortic stenosis

It should be noted that a defect occurring between the atria is termed an atrial septal defect and one between the ventricles, a ventricular septal defect. Normally, the pressure on the left side of the heart is higher than on the right side and blood will pass from left to right through the defect. If the pressure in the pulmonary artery increases (pulmonary hypertension), the flow is reversed and cyanosis occurs.

## Cyanotic Group

### TETRALOGY OF FALLOT

The tetralogy consists of pulmonary stenosis, ventricular septal defect, overriding of the aorta so that it lies over both ventricles, and right ventricular hypertrophy. As a result of the pulmonary stenosis, pressure increases in the right side of the heart and venous blood passes into the aorta.

CLINICAL FEATURES. The patient is cyanosed from shortly after birth with associated clubbing of the fingers. The patient experiences dyspnea and, when resting, adopts a squatting position characteristic of this condition.

TREATMENT is surgical.

## Acyanotic Group

### PERSISTENT DUCTUS ARTERIOSUS

The ductus joining the left pulmonary artery and the aorta normally closes at birth or soon afterwards. If it persists, there is a shunt from the aorta to the pulmonary artery resulting in an increase in pulmonary artery flow and in the output of the left ventricle.

CLINICAL FEATURES. Subacute bacterial endocarditis develops in some cases. Because of the increased work of the left ventricle, cardiac failure is another complication. There is a collapsing pulse with a low diastolic pressure. Typically, a "machinery murmur" exists and is best heard in the second left intercostal space.

TREATMENT is the surgical closure of the ductus.

### ATRIAL SEPTAL DEFECT

This condition may produce no symptoms until middle age when it usually presents as cardiac failure.

TREATMENT. Surgical repair of the defect if possible.

### VENTRICULAR SEPTAL DEFECT

A small defect may produce no symptoms (Maladie de Roger). In some cases, bacterial endocarditis occurs (see p. 50). If the defect is large, the output of the left ventricle is increased and heart failure may result. More commonly, pulmonary hypertension develops and results in a right-to-left shunt with consequent cyanosis.

TREATMENT. The defect is closed in selected cases.

### COARCTATION OF THE AORTA

In this condition, narrowing of the aorta, usually distal to the origin of the left subclavian artery, occurs. This results in the formation of an extensive collateral circulation.

CLINICAL FEATURES. Many patients have no symptoms. Some develop hypertension and some heart failure; in others, a subarachnoid hemorrhage may occur due to rupture of an aneurysm of the circle of Willis which is present in about 15 percent of cases. The blood pressure rises in the arms while it remains normal in the legs. The femoral pulses are either absent or barely palpable. A radiograph of the chest will often show notching of the ribs due to pressure from the enlarged intercostal arteries.

TREATMENT. The narrowed portion of the aorta is resected.

## PULMONARY STENOSIS

CLINICAL FEATURES. In mild cases there may be no symptoms and the condition may be found on routine examination. Severe cases usually have right ventricular enlargement and develop cardiac failure by early adult life.

TREATMENT. The treatment of severe pulmonary stenosis is surgical widening of the valve.

## CONGENITAL AORTIC STENOSIS

Aortic stenosis may be of congenital origin or may result from rheumatic involvement or extensive atheroma of the aortic valve. When rheumatic in origin it is frequently associated with mitral stenosis. Atheroma of the aortic valve is more common in the elderly. All three forms of aortic stenosis have similar clinical features.

CLINICAL FEATURES. When the disorder is mild, no symptoms may be present but in most cases the strain on the left ventricle produces first hypertrophy and then dilatation and failure. The narrowed aortic valve results in a small pulse and reduction of cardiac output. This may lead to fainting on effort and angina.

TREATMENT. Mild cases require no treatment but the patient should avoid undue physical effort. Extraction of teeth or scaling require antibiotic cover (see under Prophylaxis of Subacute Bacterial Endocarditis, p. 51). In severe cases widening of the aortic valve is performed or, if there is aortic regurgitation, some form of artificial valve may be inserted.

## CONGESTIVE HEART FAILURE

Heart failure occurs when the ventricles fail to maintain an adequate output of blood for the needs of the body. The result is congestion in the pulmonary or the systemic circulation or both. The manifestations of pulmonary vascular engorgement commonly are referred to as *left heart failure* and those of systemic venous and capillary engorgement as *right heart failure*.

### Left Ventricular Failure

The chief causes of left ventricular failure are:
1. Hypertension
2. Coronary artery disease
3. Aortic valvular disease

When the left ventricle is required to do increased work, it responds by undergoing hypertrophy and this process enables it for a time to maintain an adequate circulation. Eventually, however, the ventricle can no longer maintain an adequate output and pressure rises in the left atrium and the pulmonary veins leading to pulmonary venous congestion and edema.

CLINICAL FEATURES. Left ventricular failure may develop gradually or happen suddenly; sudden onset is most commonly due to coronary thrombosis. At first the patient may require two or more pillows to prevent his difficulty in breathing when lying flat (orthopnea). Later he awakens from sleep fighting for breath (cardiac asthma) and may expectorate copious amounts of blood-tinged sputum.

TREATMENT. The patient is kept upright with pillows behind the back. Morphine (intramuscularly) and aminophylline (intravenously) are given. Digitalis is given to those patients who have not been digitalized.

### Right Ventricular Failure

The chief causes of right ventricular failure are:
1. Left ventricular failure
2. Mitral valvular disease
3. Pulmonary heart disease
4. Certain types of congenital heart disease
5. Thyrotoxicosis

CLINICAL FEATURES. The main finding in right ventricular failure is *distended neck veins*. In a normal subject reclining at 30°, the neck veins are empty above the clavicles. Distention of the liver with blood follows right ventricular failure and the *liver on palpation is enlarged and tender*. *Cyanosis* is common, partly because of poor oxygenation of the blood passing through the edematous lungs and partly because of peripheral stagnation. Right ventricular failure is usually seen in patients who already suffer dyspnea and orthopnea from pulmonary congestion due to left ventricular failure or mitral valvular disease and is then often called congestive cardiac failure.

TREATMENT. Many right ventricular and congestive failure patients prefer to sleep in a high-backed armchair. A light diet is given with salt restricted to one gram per day. Digitalis is administered and results in a rise in cardiac output and a fall in venous pressure. Diuretics assist in reducing the extracellular fluid. The patient is sedated and oxygen is administered when there is cyanosis.

### SHOCK

In shock, there is circulatory collapse frequently associated with a reduction in the venous return and resulting in a deficiency of blood to the periphery. It may follow such conditions as severe trauma, hemorrhage, major surgery and myocardial infarction.

MECHANISM OF SHOCK. Shock may result from:
1. Decreased blood volume

2. Peripheral vasodilatation

3. Myocardial failure or a combination of these factors

Decreased blood volume (hypovolemia) may be caused by hemorrhage or by loss of plasma as in extensive burns. The reduction in venous return causes a fall in blood pressure which is corrected in part by vasoconstriction and tachycardia. The renal blood flow is diminished as a result of the vasoconstriction and leads to oliguria and, if very severe, to anuria.

Peripheral vasodilatation occurs in the common faint (syncope). As a result of emotion or exposure to warm atmosphere, a vasovagal reflex occurs producing bradycardia, vasodilatation and a consequent fall in blood pressure. The latter causes an abrupt reduction in cerebral blood flow and the patient falls to the ground; when the patient is in the horizontal position, the cerebral anemia is corrected.

In myocardial infarction the muscular contractility of the heart is impaired so that cardiac output is decreased and arterial pressure falls; central venous pressure, however, may be normal or even elevated.

CLINICAL FEATURES. The patient is pale, sweating and restless. The pulse is rapid and in some cases may be barely palpable.

TREATMENT. In the early stages, syncope can be relieved by placing the patient's head between his legs. The patient may be placed in the supine position and his legs elevated to facilitate return of venous blood to the heart.

Shock due to hemorrhage can be corrected by transfusion of whole blood carefully matched and cross matched and by control of hemorrhage. Burn shock is treated by transfusion of plasma or whole blood. Restlessness and pain are controlled by a subcutaneous injection of morphine or meperidine. Vasopressors such as metaraminol intravenously are of value in increasing the systolic blood pressure.

## DISORDERS OF THE HEART BEAT

### Normal Mechanism

In the normal heart, the stimulus for the heart beat arises in the sinoatrial node, the heart's pacemaker. From here, the impulse spreads through the atrial musculature as a wave of electrical discharges which is followed by contraction. When the impulse reaches the atrioventricular node, it is delayed momentarily. It then passes down the bundle branches, the Purkinje system and then through the musculature, resulting in ventricular contraction. The electrocardiogram provides a graphic record of the electrical activity of the heart and is necessary for accurate diagnosis of cardiac conditions.

The first heart sound occurs at the beginning of ventricular systole. It is caused by the closure of the tricuspid and mitral valves. The second sound marks the beginning of ventricular diastole and is caused by the closure of aortic and pulmonary valves.

As a result of congenital cardiac anomalies or of diseases such as rheumatic fever in which the cardiac valves may be involved, *murmurs* are produced which may be systolic or diastolic in timing. *Thrills* are palpable murmurs.

## Premature Beats

Premature beats are the result of an abnormal stimulus arising in either an atrium, a ventricle or at the atrioventricular node. Occasional premature beats are common occurrences and often are experienced by the normal individual. In persons with heart disease, however, they occur frequently.

## Paroxysmal Tachycardia

Paroxysmal tachycardia may arise as the result of an ectopic focus in the atrium or in the ventricles. The heart rate is usually between 160 and 200 beats per minute. In paroxysmal atrial tachycardia, the rhythm is regular and not affected by exercise. The beginning and ending of a paroxysm are abrupt. Pressure on the carotid sinus may cause the heart rate to revert to normal. An occasional attack of paroxysmal atrial tachycardia does not in itself indicate organic heart disease. The patient with ventricular tachycardia, on the other hand, has a disturbance which usually indicates heart disease.

## Atrial Flutter

In atrial flutter, which is nearly always associated with heart disease, there is a regular rapid beat, varying usually from 250 to 350 per minute. The ventricles are unable to respond at this rate so that there is usually some degree of partial atrioventricular block, the ventricles only responding to every second, third or fourth atrial contraction. The patient typically presents himself because of uncomfortable and alarming palpitation, breathlessness and weakness. Atrial flutter can be distinguished from atrial fibrillation by carotid sinus stimulation which will cut the heart rate of the former in half.

## Atrial Fibrillation

In atrial fibrillation the atrial rate is irregular and between 400 and 500 per minute; atrial contraction is not coordinated.

Atrial fibrillation is usually associated with heart disease such as mitral stenosis, thyrotoxicosis, coronary artery disease and hypertension.

CLINICAL FEATURES. Usually the patient complains of palpitations and may notice the irregularity of the pulse. Occasionally the onset is more dramatic with fainting and collapse followed possibly by acute cardiac failure. The diagnosis can be confirmed by feeling the pulse, which is characteristically completely irregular in force and rhythm.

TREATMENT. Digitalis is the drug of choice in most cases. In some patients normal sinus rhythm can be restored by direct current shock (cardioversion).

## Heart Block

In some patients, conduction through the atrioventricular node fails and may result in sudden death. In others, after a variable period of asystole, the ventricle begins to contract automatically. If the ectopic focus is high in the ventricular muscle, the heart rate is between 50 and 70 per minute. If the focus is low, the rate is slow and fixed. On occasion, the rate is so slow that an adequate cardiac output is not generated.

CLINICAL FEATURES. The patient is bedridden because of weakness, cerebral anoxia and congestive heart failure If the ventricle should suddenly stop beating, the clinical picture is that of cerebral anoxia, syncope and convulsions—the Stokes-Adams attack. Congenital complete heart block is usually asymptomatic.

TREATMENT. A permanent cardiac pacemaker can be implanted and will relieve the symptoms.

## THE BLOOD PRESSURE

The height of the blood pressure depends on the cardiac output and the peripheral resistance to blood flow. The systolic pressure is the maximum pressure developed on the ejection of blood from the left ventricle into the arteries. The lowest pressure is the diastolic and is a measure of the peripheral resistance.

In measuring the blood pressure by the auscultatory method, the systolic pressure is taken at the point when beats become audible. As the mercury continues to fall, the sound of the beats becomes louder, then gradually diminishes until a point is reached at which there is a sudden, marked diminution in intensity. At a point five to ten mms. lower, the beats disappear altogether. The American Heart Association recommends that the point of disappearance of the sounds be used as the most reliable index of diastolic pressure.

The average blood pressure is about 120/80 at the age of twenty rising to 160/90 at the age of sixty. The upper limit of normal is taken as a diastolic pressure of 90 mm. and readings above this are classified as hypertension. The differences between the systolic and diastolic pressure is the pulse pressure, e.g. $160 - 90 = 70$ mm.

## Hypertension

Hypertension, elevation of the blood pressure, may be classified as follows:

1. Essential hypertension
   a. Benign
   b. Malignant
2. Hypertension associated with renal disease

3. Other rare causes
   a. Coarctation of the aorta
   b. Hypertension associated with endocrine disease
      Cushing's syndrome
      Pheochromocytoma

## ESSENTIAL HYPERTENSION

Essential hypertension is the most common form of hypertension. The cause is unknown. In malignant hypertension, which is less frequent than the benign type, the diastolic pressure is markedly raised (usually from 130 to 160 mm. Hg.).

CLINICAL FEATURES. The patient may remain symptomless for years. Ultimately, the cardiovascular system and the kidneys become involved.

THE HEART. Because the heart is working against increased resistance, the left ventricle enlarges and may ultimately fail resulting in dyspnea on effort and paroxysmal dyspnea at night. Eventually, the left ventricular failure may progress to right ventricular failure with distended neck veins and peripheral edema.

THE BLOOD VESSELS. The medium-sized arteries, e.g. the radial, thicken. In addition, the arteries of the retina are involved.

CEREBRAL ARTERIES. In severe hypertension, involvement of the cerebral arteries leads to headaches which are usually worse in the morning. Cerebral edema may also occur resulting in *hypertensive encephalopathy* with severe headaches, fits, unconsciousness and nerve palsies. A common complication is cerebral hemorrhage.

THE KIDNEY. Renal involvement is more marked in malignant than in benign hypertension. In the former, there are marked changes in the blood vessels of the kidney leading to progressive decrease in renal function and death may occur from renal failure.

TREATMENT. Sedatives and hypotensive drugs are employed.

### Hypotension

Hypotension, low blood pressure, results either from a decrease in cardiac output or from a decrease in peripheral resistance. The cardiac output is decreased in Addison's disease, myocardial infarction, myocarditis and following hemorrhage.

Hypotension due to decreased peripheral resistance may occur in pneumonia, septicemia and acute adrenal insufficiency (Waterhouse-Friderichsen syndrome).

TREATMENT. This depends entirely on the cause. When hypotension is due to cardiac disease, treatment is directed towards relief of the cardiac lesion. Extensive blood loss is corrected by blood transfusion. Hypotension resulting from severe infections demands antibiotic therapy. The treatment of Addison's disease is discussed on page 138.

# RHEUMATIC HEART DISEASE

## Acute Rheumatic Fever

Acute rheumatic fever is a disease affecting connective tissue, particularly that of the heart and its valves and the joints. Children between the ages of eight and fifteen are most commonly affected, especially those in the lower economic groups.

ETIOLOGY. The disease usually occurs two or three weeks after a sore throat due to infection with a $\beta$-hemolytic streptococcus (Lancefield Group A). It is thought likely that the lesions represent an allergic reaction to exotoxins from the hemolytic streptococcus in a patient who has been previously sensitized.

CLINICAL FEATURES. Typically, the illness starts suddenly with fever, pain, stiffness and sometimes swelling in a large joint such as the knee or elbow. Characteristically the pain flits from joint to joint. Rheumatic nodules occur over the elbows, wrists and shins. They are about the size of a pea and are not attached to the overlying skin. Skin rashes are sometimes seen.

In a percentage of cases, the rheumatic process is insidious and may be overlooked.

Cardiac involvement occurs and lesions known as Aschoff nodes may occur in the myocardium. These consist of a central area of necrotic collagen surrounded by a zone of inflammatory cells—polymorphs, macrophages, giant cells and later fibroblasts.

The most important lesion of rheumatic fever is that which involves the valves. Inflammation (valvulitis) leads to swelling and deposition of small thrombi (vegetations) on the cusps, especially along the lines of their closure. While most other lesions of rheumatic fever undergo resolution, those of the valves do not. They tend to progress to a state of chronic inflammation and the cusps become thickened, fibrosed and contracted. Adjacent cusps adhere to each other rendering the orifice stenotic while the rigid leaflets and thickened, contracted chordae tendineae lead to regurgitation. If the aortic valve is affected, it is usually both stenosed and incompetent. Mitral stenosis is the most common valvular lesion of rheumatic heart disease. Blood is dammed back in the left atrium and pulmonary venous congestion follows. In mitral stenosis, the left ventricle is under no strain and is, therefore, small but should there be mitral regurgitation or an aortic lesion, the left ventricle becomes enlarged and may subsequently fail.

LABORATORY DIAGNOSIS. The blood shows a moderate leukocytosis with some anemia and a raised erythrocyte sedimentation rate. The anti-streptolysin titer in the blood is raised.

TREATMENT. Rest is essential. Penicillin is administered throughout the illness. In penicillin-sensitive patients erythromycin is given. The specific drugs used in the relief of rheumatic fever are the salicylates. Cortisone is used for patients who fail to respond to the usual treatment.

## ARTERIOSCLEROTIC HEART DISEASE

The myocardium is supplied by blood through the two coronary arteries. These vessels are particularly liable to be affected by atheroma which causes a narrowing of their lumina and subsequent myocardial ischemia.

### Gradual Coronary Occlusion

The patient begins to notice pain in the chest on exercise (angina pectoris). Characteristically the pain is felt beneath the sternum and is crushing in character. It may spread into the neck or down the left arm. It comes on with exercise and is relieved by rest.

TREATMENT. Glyceryl trinitrate is chewed or sucked and will relieve the pain within two to three minutes.

DENTAL MANAGEMENT OF A PATIENT WITH ANGINA PECTORIS. The patient should be routinely sedated as emotional stress is not well-tolerated. About five minutes before starting local anesthesia, the patient should be premedicated with nitroglycerin sublingually.

### Sudden Coronary Occlusion

Coronary atheroma is particularly liable to be complicated by thrombosis which leads to a sudden complete occlusion of the lumen, thus cutting off the blood supply to an area of heart muscle. Acute ischemia may cause sudden death. If the patient survives, the ischemic muscles undergo necrosis and an infarct is produced. Later the dead muscle is replaced by a fibrous scar.

CLINICAL FEATURES. The onset is sudden and the pain resembles that of angina pectoris except that it is not relieved by rest and persists for several hours. On examination, the patient is anxious, pale, sweating and with a rapid pulse and low blood pressure. Cardiac arrhythmias may occur with coronary thrombosis, one of the most common being ventricular extrasystoles; these may herald the onset of a dangerous ventricular tachycardia or even ventricular fibrillation.

During the first week, there is often a rise in temperature, a polymorphonuclear leukocytosis and a rise in the sedimentation rate, all indications of the inflammatory reaction around the damaged myocardium.

Necrotic muscle releases its enzymes into the blood and a rise in the levels of serum GOT (glutamic oxaloacetic transaminase) and serum GPT (glutamic pyruvic transaminase) occur in myocardial infarction. An EKG is used to confirm the diagnosis.

TREATMENT. Bed rest for about four weeks. Severe pain is relieved by morphine. Anticoagulants are used in "bad risk" cases particularly in those patients who have had a previous infarct.

## Complications of Myocardial Infarction

### PERICARDITIS

This occurs if the infarct involves the pericardial surface.

### MURAL THROMBOSIS

Mural thrombosis is seen if the infarct involves the endocardium. Portions of thrombus may break off and emboli may occur in systemic organs like the brain and kidney.

### RUPTURE

Occasionally, the necrotic muscle ruptures and this causes bleeding into the pericardial cavity and sudden death. Both this complication and systemic embolism are likely to occur at the end of the first week.

About 70 percent of patients with coronary thrombosis survive their first attack. The infarct organizes and a fibrous scar is produced which may later bulge. The aneurysm of the left ventricle so formed may ultimately rupture but this is an uncommon event. Usually the patient is left with some degree of heart failure and may have further episodes of coronary thrombosis.

DENTAL MANAGEMENT. It is wiser to avoid prolonged dental treatment for at least six months after coronary thrombosis.

## BACTERIAL ENDOCARDITIS

In bacterial endocarditis, bacterial invasion of a heart valve or of the endocardium takes place. Bacterial endocarditis may be classified into two types depending on the virulence of the invading organism—acute bacterial endocarditis and subacute bacterial endocarditis.

### Acute Bacterial Endocarditis

During an acute septicemia with virulent organisms such as *Staphylococcus aureus*, gonococcus or *Streptococcus pyogenes*, previously normal heart valves may be invaded and rapidly destroyed. The clinical picture is that of an acute septicemia and the condition is frequently fatal. (See Treatment of Bacterial Endocarditis below.)

### Subacute Bacterial Endocarditis

The most common causative organism of this condition is *Streptococcus viridans*. Other organisms which have been incriminated are *Streptococcus faecalis*, coagulase-negative staphylococci and anaerobic streptococci. The bacteria settle on a valve previously damaged by rheumatic fever or on congenital cardiac defects such as ventricular septal defect, persistent ductus arteriosus and bicuspid aortic valve.

The bacteria enter the bloodstream during dental extractions or in the course of an operation on the intestinal tract. After settling on the damaged valve or congenital cardiac defect, the bacteria cause an inflammatory reaction which is followed by deposits of fibrin and the formation of a vegetation that often spreads from the valve to the adjacent endocardium.

CLINICAL FEATURES. An unexplained fever or period of ill health in a patient with a history of rheumatic fever is suggestive of subacute bacterial endocarditis. Recent dental treatment precedes an attack in fifty percent of cases.

Malaise, anorexia, weight loss, excessive perspiration and shivering at night are common symptoms. Anemia develops within one or two weeks of the onset of symptoms and, in addition, the skin has a generalized brown pigmentation, "café au lait" appearance. Clubbing of the fingers occurs. Emboli originating with the heart may lodge in the skin causing small, tender, red, slightly raised areas found on the pads of the fingers. In the small vessels under the nails, emboli may lodge and give rise to multiple capillary hemorrhages (splinter hemorrhages). Red cells may appear in the urine as a result of focal embolic glomerulonephritis, "flea-bitten kidney." In the retina, emboli may produce typical hemorrhages. Larger vessels may be destroyed causing major infarcts in the liver, spleen, brain, intestines or limbs.

As a result of the chronic septicemia, the spleen is usually enlarged. Infarction may cause pain in the splenic area. The heart shows signs of the underlying valve lesion and rarely, changes in the character of the murmurs can be detected. Heart failure may develop.

LABORATORY DIAGNOSIS.

1. Blood culture is essential for diagnosis and the choice of antibiotic is made following isolation of the causative organism.

2. The peripheral blood shows an elevated sedimentation rate, progressive normocytic normochromic anemia and a mild leukocytosis.

3. The urine contains red cells on microscopy.

PROPHYLAXIS. Prophylactic antibiotics are given to cover dental extractions and scaling and tonsillectomy in patients with cardiac lesions.

For dental therapy, 600,000 units crystalline penicillin combined with 600,000 units procaine penicillin given intramuscularly one hour before the operation, continuing with procaine penicillin 600,000 units daily for two days is recommended. For patients sensitive to penicillin, sodium cephalothin (Keflin) 500 mg. administered intramuscularly immediately prior to dental extraction followed by oral erythromycin 250 mg. q.i.d. can be employed.

TREATMENT OF BACTERIAL ENDOCARDITIS. The selection of the antibiotic used is dependent on the organism isolated on blood culture. Bactericidal antibiotics are more effective than bacteriostatic drugs and must be used in high dosage and for at least six weeks. Penicillin is usually the drug of choice for *Streptococcus viridans* infection and very large doses of penicillin with some other bactericidal antibiotic such as streptomycin or ampicillin are used for *Streptococcus faecalis* infections. When penicillin is used, the intramuscular route is preferred for dosages up to 20 mega units a day.  Doses of penicillin in excess of this amount are usually given by continuous intravenous infusion because of the severe local inflammatory response to intramuscular injection of large quantities.  Cephaloridine has been used in penicillin-sensitive individuals although cross-reactions have been reported to cephaloridine in some penicillin-sensitive patients.

## THE DENTAL MANAGEMENT OF PATIENTS WITH CARDIOVASCULAR PROBLEMS

Apprehension, worry and long, fatiguing dental procedures must be minimized in those patients with cardiovascular problems.  These factors stimulate the discharge of epinephrine and norepinephrine into the circulation and may give rise to an elevation in the blood pressure and heart rate and to an anginal attack.  If a local anesthetic solution containing epinephrine is injected slowly and extravascularly, there is no danger as the epinephrine is present in too small a concentration to have a significant deleterious effect.  To prevent intravascular injection, an aspirating syringe should be used.

Care must be taken in prescribing sedative drugs when the patient is already receiving phenothiazines, antihistamines and rauwolfia drugs as potentiation and prolongation of action may occur.  In patients who are receiving phenothiazines or one of the antihypertensive agents such as hydralazine (Apresoline), guanethidine (Ismelin), methyldopa (Aldomet) or the rauwolfia alkaloids, the addition of sedatives may bring about dangerous hypotensive episodes or postural hypotension.

### Vasodilator and Antihypertensive Agents

Glyceryl trinitrate is prescribed for the treatment of angina pectoris. Because of its vasodilator effect, an abrupt fall in blood pressure may ensue and result in fainting.

Epinephrine should *not* be used for treatment of vasomotor collapse occurring in patients receiving tranquilizers, particularly phenothiazine.

The antihypertensive drugs may cause nausea and vomiting.  In addition, hypertensive patients under treatment with these drugs may develop postural hypotension or syncope more readily than the normal patient. Many of these drugs potentiate barbiturate sedation and anesthesia and, as a result, general anesthetics may produce episodes of hypotension.

Morphine or meperidine should not be administered to patients who have been treated for hypertension with a monoamine oxidase inhibitor. These drugs must be discontinued for two weeks prior to operation.  In addition, local anesthetic solutions containing epinephrine are contraindicated in patients receiving monoamine oxidase inhibitors as a profound rise of blood pressure may occur.

## Cardiac Glycosides

Any patient who is taking cardiac glycosides and who has resumed normal activities since digitalization is a good risk for dental care. If, however, the patient complains of dyspnea during his usual activities, inability to climb stairs without resting, swelling of the ankles or nocturnal dyspnea, he should be re-evaluated by his physician.

Some patients who are receiving digitalis preparations over long periods develop a tendency towards nausea and vomiting. For this reason, care must be taken during general anesthesia to avoid stimulation of the vomiting reflex and possible aspiration of vomitus.

## Diuretic Agents

Mercurial diuretics which are prescribed for cardiac and renal edema may result in mercurial stomatitis as a reaction to their mercury content. Acetazolamide (Diamox) which is also used for its diuretic effect and in the treatment of glaucoma may sometimes cause facial paresthesia.

# CARDIOPULMONARY RESUSCITATION

Cardiac arrest may occur in patients with a previous history of cardiac disease or it may arise as a result of a systemic reaction to the injection of local anesthetics, antibiotics or other drugs (anaphylactic shock) or as the result of general anesthesia. The heart may stop completely (asystole) or ventricular fibrillation may occur during the course of which the heart cannot maintain an adequate circulation to the brain and other vital organs. A heart which is in asystole may be restarted by external cardiac massage. However, to restore a normal rhythm in ventricular fibrillation a defibrillator is essential. The purpose of cardiopulmonary resuscitation in ventricular fibrillation is to maintain an adequate blood supply to the brain and vital organs until a defibrillator can be obtained.

## Steps in Cardiopulmonary Resuscitation

1. Cardiopulmonary resuscitation is best performed with the patient on the floor or some hard surface to provide adequate support during sternal compression.

2. Mouth-to-mouth insufflation is begun after clearing the airway and hyperextending the head. Ventilation with 100 percent oxygen is the most satisfactory but may not always be available. Twelve respirations per minute are preferable for adults but for the single operator eight will suffice. In children the lungs should be inflated 20 times per minute.

3. Sternal compression is begun at a rate of 60–80 per minute and continued until an effective cardiac mechanism is restored.

These are emergency measures which are later followed by:

4. An intravenous drip is started and sodium bicarbonate 3.75 Gm. per 50 ml. is given immediately and every five minutes during resuscitation to combat acidosis.

5. Intravenous epinephrine 0.5 to 1.0 ml. of a 1:1000 dilution is given early and repeatedly before electrical depolarization. Calcium chloride (10 ml. of 10-percent solution) is also useful in restoring myocardial tone, pulse pressure and cardiac output.

6. Electrical depolarization is given.

# DISEASES OF THE BLOOD VESSELS

## Diseases of the Arteries

Diseases of the arteries may be subdivided into:
1. Chronic obliterative arterial disease due to:
   a. Atherosclerosis
   b. Buerger's disease (thromboangiitis obliterans)
2. Acute obstruction to the arterial circulation by embolism or thrombosis
3. Raynaud's phenomenon

### ATHEROSCLEROSIS

In this condition, which occurs most commonly over the age of 50, fatty material accumulates in the intima and fibrosis is associated. It occurs most frequently in the arteries supplying the lower limbs.

CLINICAL FEATURES. The earliest symptom is intermittent claudication which is cramp-like pain occurring usually in the calf or more rarely in the thigh, causing the patient to limp. It may be brought on by walking and is quickly relieved by rest. In severe cases, pain may occur at rest and may keep the patient awake at night.

Examination shows pallor of the limb and absent or reduced pulses. If the circulation to the limb is severely impaired, gangrene may occur.

TREATMENT. Care of the feet is essential to prevent gangrene. Vaso-dilators are used to improve the circulation. Tobacco reduces peripheral blood flow and the patient should stop smoking. Arterial grafting may be necessary, and amputation is indicated in cases of gangrene.

### BUERGER'S DISEASE

This disease affects both the arteries and the veins of the legs and causes ischemia. It occurs almost exclusively in men and usually starts between the ages of 25 and 45.

CLINICAL FEATURES. Intermittent claudication is the common symptom.

TREATMENT. The treatment is the same as for atherosclerosis.

### ACUTE ARTERIAL OBSTRUCTION

Acute arterial obstruction may result from a thrombus or an embolus. Thrombosis may occur on an atheromatous plaque. Emboli arise from the left side of the heart, usually in a patient with mitral stenosis or subacute bacterial endocarditis.

CLINICAL FEATURES. The onset is sudden with severe pain, pallor, coldness, loss of sensation and weakness in the affected limb. The arterial pulses disappear below the level of the obstruction.

Within six hours of the obstruction, embolectomy may be performed. If not, anticoagulants are given and the limb is kept cool to reduce its oxygen requirements. Amputation may be required.

## RAYNAUD'S PHENOMENON

Raynaud's phenomenon is produced by spasm of the digital arteries and may be the result of a number of causes:
1. Hypersensitivity of the digital vessels to cold (Raynaud's disease)
2. Autoimmune disorders, especially lupus erythematosus and scleroderma
3. Occupational in people handling vibrating tools
4. Other arterial diseases, atherosclerosis, Buerger's disease

CLINICAL FEATURES. Raynaud's phenomenon is more common in young women who complain of cold, white fingers, particularly on exposure to cold. In severe cases gangrene of the tips of the fingers may develop. Occasionally the tip of the nose and the toes are affected.

TREATMENT. The patient should be kept as warm as possible. Vasodilators are prescribed; in severe cases sympathectomy is indicated.

### Diseases of the Veins

Venous thrombosis is not uncommon and there are two varieties:
1. Phlebothrombosis
2. Thrombophlebitis

## PHLEBOTHROMBOSIS

In this condition, extensive thrombosis and clot formation occur in the veins of the calf. It is essentially due to stasis and occurs wherever a patient is put to bed, especially if he is elderly, if the heart is failing or if he is shocked or has suffered severe trauma or hemorrhage.

CLINICAL FEATURES. The symptoms are often slight. There is little pain in the limb but direct squeezing pressure on the calf muscles may elicit tenderness. The ankle may swell slightly. Frequently the first indication of phlebothrombosis is the occurrence of pulmonary embolism.

TREATMENT. Anticoagulants. The patient is gotten out of bed as soon as possible.

COMPLICATIONS. Small emboli may lodge in the lungs and may sometimes produce infarction. A more serious complication is massive pulmonary embolism which produces sudden death. This usually occurs seven to ten days after an injury or operation.

## THROMBOPHLEBITIS

Inflammation of the vessel wall may follow the injection of irritant chemicals such as anesthetic agents or may be the result of spread of infection from an adjacent staphylococcal abscess. Thrombosis occurs in the area of damage but as stasis is not present, extensive propagation of the clot does not occur. The thrombosis is, therefore, relatively localized and firmly adherent.

CLINICAL FEATURES. There may be fever, slight elevation of the pulse and a leukocytosis. The patient is usually restless; there is swelling of the extremity and tenderness over the involved vein.

TREATMENT. In mild thrombophlebitis heparin is administered, the limb is bandaged to support the veins and the patient is allowed out of bed. In thrombophlebitis associated with pain, fever and tachycardia, heparin is administered together with sedation and the patient is kept in bed.

## GENERAL REFERENCES

*Accepted Dental Therapeutics*, 33rd ed., Chicago, American Dental Association, 1970.

Fleming, J. S. and Braimbridge, M. V.: *Lecture Notes on Cardiology*, Oxford, Blackwell Scientific Publications, 1967.

Houston, J. C., Joiner, C. L., and Trounce, J. R.: *A Short Textbook of Medicine*, 3rd ed. Philadelphia, Lippincott, 1968.

Talso, P. J. and Remenchik, A. P.: *Internal Medicine Based on Mechanisms of Disease*, St. Louis, Mosby, 1968.

## SUGGESTED READING

Fay, J. T.: Dental procedures for the patient with cardiovascular disease. JADA, *78*, 105, 1969.

Myall, R. W. T. and Gregory, H. S.: Current trends in the prevention of bacterial endocarditis in susceptible patients receiving dental care. Oral Surg., *28*, 813, 1969.

## CHAPTER 5

# DISEASES OF THE KIDNEY

The kidney has two main functions:

1. It excretes the end products of metabolism such as urea, uric acid and creatinine. Many drugs are also excreted by this route.

2. It maintains the pH and volume of the tissue fluids.

In the passage of the glomerular filtrate down the renal tubules, 80 percent of the water is reabsorbed in the proximal segment. In the loop of Henle the concentration of the urine increases progressively as it passes down the tubule towards the renal medulla and then decreases once again as the tubular fluid returns to the cortex. This mechanism is described as the principle of countercurrent multiplication concentration. In the distal convoluted tubule and the collecting duct, the rate of urine formation is controlled by the level of antidiuretic hormone (ADH). Sodium reabsorption and potassium excretion in this segment is controlled by aldosterone.

## Control of Aldosterone Secretion

The kidney is believed to play a role in the control of aldosterone secretion. The juxtaglomerular apparatus in the kidney secretes renin, an enzyme which converts circulating angiotensinogen into angiotensin I which is further converted to angiotensin II. The latter is a potent vasoconstrictor and stimulates aldosterone secretion.

## Erythropoietin Production

The kidney is the site of production of erythropoietin which is essential for erythropoiesis. Excess erythropoietin may be formed and secondary polycythemia may occur in some patients where an underlying renal lesion such as a neoplasm, cyst or hydronephrosis exists.

## CLINICAL EVALUATION OF RENAL FUNCTION
### Urine Examination

Routine urinalysis should include a determination of pH and specific gravity, and a qualitative estimation of protein, glucose and acetone. If, on a random urine specimen, the specific gravity is 1.022 or greater and there is no significant glycosuria or marked proteinuria, then it is reasonable to conclude that the overall renal function is adequate.

Clean-voided specimens of urine are obtained by cleansing the external genitalia and collecting the second half of the voiding in a sterile container. In the female, vaginal contamination is prevented with a gauze tampon. The urine is then centrifuged, the supernatant discarded and the sediment resuspended in the few remaining drops of urine. Normal urine collected in this way contains no more than one or two red blood cells and one or two white blood cells and epithelial cells per high-power field. Hyaline casts resulting from the precipitation of pure protein in the renal tubules are found very occasionally in a lower-power field. In renal diseases, particularly glomerulonephritis, desquamated renal tubular epithelial cells are found in the urine.

### Other Tests of Renal Function

Urea represents the major end product of protein metabolism and is excreted through the kidneys. In patients with advanced renal disease, the level of the blood urea nitrogen provides a rough index of the impairment of the renal function. For this reason, the blood urea determination is frequently employed. The endogenous creatinine clearance and the urea clearance are the most reliable tests of glomerular function. The phenolsulfonphthalein test depends on the ability of the kidney to excrete this dye and is used in the quantitative assessment of kidney damage.

### Renal Biopsy

When the exact diagnosis is obscure, a needle biopsy of the kidney is employed and the tissue is examined with both the light and electron microscopes.

## SPECIFIC DISORDERS OF THE KIDNEY
### Glomerulonephritis

Glomerulonephritis is primarily an inflammation affecting glomerular tufts.

### ACUTE GLOMERULONEPHRITIS

CLINICAL FEATURES. Acute glomerulonephritis occurs most commonly in children and adolescents and usually follows one to three weeks after a throat infection with Group A, β-hemolytic streptococci. Only a few serologic types of group A streptococci have been implicated. The onset is fairly sudden with malaise, shivering and fever and some patients complain of pain in the loins or abdomen. The patient commonly presents with edema around the eyes and the face has a puffy appearance. The blood pressure is usually moderately raised. The urine is decreased in volume and contains red cells and protein which give it a reddish appearance.

In 80 to 90 percent of children with acute glomerulonephritis, recovery is complete and permanent. Within a few days a diuresis occurs, the edema subsides and the blood pressure falls; the entire disease lasts two to four weeks. Of the remaining 10 to 20 percent, some patients die of renal failure while the rest continue to excrete albumin in the urine.

Twenty to fifty percent of adults with acute glomerulonephritis either die during the acute episode or develop chronic kidney disease. The remainder recover.

TREATMENT. The objective of treatment is to maintain water and electrolyte balance and to provide adequate calories until there is spontaneous recovery of renal function. Salt and fluids are restricted and a diet consisting mainly of carbohydrates and fats is prescribed. Penicillin is given for ten days to eliminate all streptococci from the throat.

## CHRONIC GLOMERULONEPHRITIS

Chronic glomerulonephritis may follow an attack of acute glomerulonephritis or it may occur without any history of renal disease.

CLINICAL FEATURES. In some patients, the disease may be symptomless and abnormal urinary findings may only be found on routine physical examination. In others, the patient may complain of fatigue, anemia and breathlessness.

Ultimately the symptoms of uremia develop, often complicated by severe hypertension resulting in death.

TREATMENT. The purpose of the treatment is to maintain renal function. At least six pints of fluid daily are required. Protein is restricted in patients where the blood urea is high. If the hypertension is severe, it is treated with antihypertensive drugs.

### Pyelonephritis

Pyelonephritis is a condition in which the ureters, renal pelvis and renal parenchyma are inflamed. The disease is a major cause of renal failure and hypertension. It may occur in the acute or chronic forms. The most common infecting organism is *Escherichia coli* and this may be isolated on culture of the urine.

In children usually some underlying congenital defect of the urinary tract makes the patient susceptible to the disorder. Urinary stasis predisposes to infection, and therefore pyelonephritis occurs more frequently in pregnancy and in prostatic enlargement.

CLINICAL FEATURES. Acute pyelonephritis frequently presents with fever, pain in the flanks and tenderness with frequency, urgency and pain on micturition (dysuria). Often gastrointestinal symptoms of nausea and vomiting may dominate the picture.

Chronic pyelonephritis frequently presents with symptoms of uremia, anemia or hypertension.

TREATMENT. Where there is obstruction to the passage of urine, this is dealt with surgically. The appropriate antibiotic is administered.

### The Nephrotic Syndrome

The nephrotic syndrome is characterized by heavy proteinuria, low plasma proteins and edema. It may be a complication of glomerulonephritis or systemic diseases such as diabetes mellitus, renal amyloidosis and systemic lupus erythematosus. Nearly all the diseases causing the nephrotic syndrome produce changes in the glomerulus.

An electron micrograph of the normal human glomerulus in cross section shows the basement membrane of the capillary together with, on either side, the endothelial cell of the capillary and the epithelial cell layer which is attached to the basement membrane by extensions called foot processes (Figure 5.1).

Renal biopsy shows in the majority of cases three types of glomerular abnormality:

1. *"Minimal change."* This lesion is seen in patients with no hematuria or renal excretory impairment. It is the typical lesion of the nephrotic syndrome in childhood and accounts for about 30 percent of adult cases. Light microscopy reveals no change (Figure 5.2) but examination under the

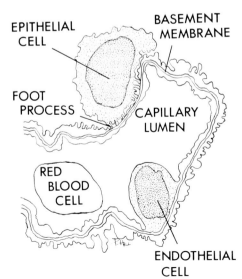

EPITHELIAL CELL

BASEMENT MEMBRANE

FOOT PROCESS

CAPILLARY LUMEN

RED BLOOD CELL

ENDOTHELIAL CELL

**Figure 5.1.** Normal glomerulus showing the foot processes of the epithelial cells and their relationship to the basement membrane. Electron microscopic appearance.

electron microscope shows basement membrane irregularity and swelling, disorganization and finally loss of the foot processes of the epithelial cells.

2. *Membranous glomerulonephritis.* This form is rare in childhood but accounts for 20 percent of adult cases. Light microscopy reveals basement membrane thickening (Figure 5.3).

3. *Proliferative glomerulonephritis.* The histologic appearances differ from slight hypercellularity of the glomerulus to epithelial crescent formation and obliteration of the glomeruli (Figure 5.4).

CLINICAL FEATURES. Proteinuria occurs until the plasma proteins fall to a low level and edema begins to appear. This is at first confined to the ankles but finally it may affect the whole body. Ultimately, renal failure develops in the majority of patients. The blood pressure and blood urea levels begin to rise, the proteinuria and edema often diminish at this stage and death ensues from renal failure.

TREATMENT. The treatment is dependent on the results of renal biopsy. Minimal change and mild proliferative glomerulonephritis are treated with steroids. Diuretics are used if steroids are not given, or if the response to steroids is delayed. When hypoproteinemia is severe, intravenous albumin may decrease the edema. A high-protein diet is given unless there is azotemia also. Intercurrent infections are controlled by antibiotics.

### Renal Failure

Renal failure is said to occur when the kidneys are unable to carry out their normal excretory functions adequately. The condition may be either acute or chronic.

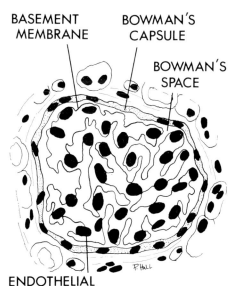

BASEMENT MEMBRANE   BOWMAN'S CAPSULE

BOWMAN'S SPACE

ENDOTHELIAL CELL

**Figure 5.2.** Normal glomerulus. Light microscopic appearance.

THICKENED
BASEMENT
MEMBRANE

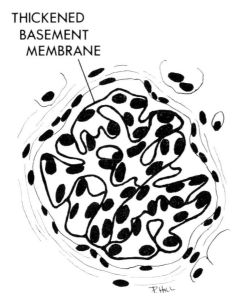

**Figure 5.3.** Membranous glomerulonephritis showing thickened basement membrane. Light microscopic
appearance.

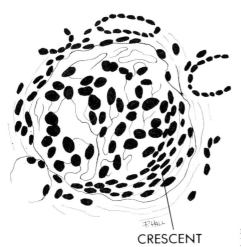

CRESCENT

**Figure 5.4.** Proliferative glomerulonephritis with crescent formation.
Light microscopic appearance.

## ACUTE RENAL FAILURE

In acute renal failure, there is sudden marked reduction in urine flow
following an episode of trauma, severe burns, a transfusion reaction or
administration of a drug. It is characterized by nitrogen retention, acidosis
and rising serum potassium.

TREATMENT. Fluid intake is restricted and glucose is given by mouth
when possible or otherwise intravenously. If the patient's condition
deteriorates, it may be necessary to employ dialysis.

## CHRONIC RENAL FAILURE

Chronic renal failure frequently follows in patients with chronic pyelonephritis, chronic glomerulonephritis and malignant hypertension. It is characterized in the advanced stage by a rising blood urea and the clinical picture of uremia. The patient at first is drowsy and then lapses into coma. Nausea, anorexia, vomiting, hiccup and diarrhea occur. Release of urea into the gastrointestinal tract gives the breath a uriniferous odor and causes stomatitis, hematemesis or melena. Hypertension is nearly always found in chronic renal failure. A progressive anemia occurs. Urea is excreted through the sebaceous glands and may crystallize on the skin as "urea frost." A small proportion of cases of chronic renal failure show widespread bone decalcification, renal osteodystrophy.

TREATMENT. In the early stages of chronic renal failure, a low-protein diet is given. If hypertension is present, this is treated with sodium restriction and hypotensive drugs. Patients with renal osteodystrophy are treated with large doses of vitamin D. As the disease advances, renal dialysis using the artificial kidney or kidney transplantation is needed.

### GENERAL REFERENCES

Douglas, A. P. and Kerr, D. N. S.: *A Short Textbook of Kidney Disease*, Philadelphia, J. B. Lippincott, 1968.

Kark, R. M., Lawrence, J. R., Pollak, V. E., Pirani, C. L., Muehrcke, R. C., and Silva, H.: *A Primer of Urinalysis*, 2nd ed., New York, Hoeber, 1963.

**CHAPTER 6**

# DISEASES OF THE GASTROINTESTINAL TRACT

The gastrointestinal tract is concerned with the digestion of food and the absorption through the intestinal wall of the products of digestion together with water, vitamins and inorganic salts. Conditions which affect the gastrointestinal tract include congenital anomalies, infections, ulcerations and neoplasms.

## THE ORAL CAVITY

Within the oral cavity conditions of both local and systemic origin occur. The oral mucosa in health varies in color from pink to pinkish-red in the white races. In the colored races, pigmentation is a normal finding and is variable in amount. Variations in color of the oral mucosa include pallor, erythema, cyanosis, jaundice, white patches and pigmentation.

The geriatric patient may frequently complain of soreness of the mouth and examination of the oral cavity may reveal a mucosa which is less resilient than normal and is referred to as atrophic. In the elderly female atrophy of the mucosa is believed to be related to involution of the ovaries although there may be other causes such as poor nutrition.

### Oral Ulceration

Ulceration of the oral mucosa is a fairly common problem confronting the dentist. There are a number of causes of oral ulceration and these are dealt with in textbooks of oral medicine and oral pathology.

It must be stressed that in the investigation of the etiology of an oral ulcer it may be necessary to take a smear from the ulcer for bacteriologic examination to exclude an infective cause. Venipuncture may be required in order to carry out a complete blood count (CBC) to exclude a blood dyscrasia or to perform a VDRL (Venereal Disease Research Laboratory) test to exclude syphilis. Exfoliative cytologic examination is useful in determining whether an ulcer is herpetic or carcinomatous. Biopsy is essential to establish the definitive diagnosis.

### White Lesions of the Oral Cavity

A number of different types of white lesions occur in the oral cavity; some are entirely benign and others are malignant or may undergo malignant change. They are adequately dealt with in textbooks of oral pathology and oral medicine.

All white lesions of the oral cavity with the possible exception of acute candidiasis (thrush) should be biopsied to establish a definitive diagnosis. In the case of acute candidiasis, a smear of the lesion and culture on to Sabouraud's medium or corn meal agar will enable a diagnosis to be made.

## THE ESOPHAGUS

A common symptom of diseases of the esophagus is dysphagia or difficulty in swallowing. This may result from anatomic defects such as achalasia of the cardia, diseases of the central nervous system and carcinoma of the esophagus.

### Peptic Esophagitis and Hiatus Hernia

The squamous epithelium of the esophagus is not designed to resist the digestive action of acid gastric juice and it frequently becomes inflamed and eroded in patients with gastroesophageal reflux. Such reflux occurs particularly, but not exclusively, in association with hiatus hernia. In the latter condition herniation of the stomach occurs through the esophageal hiatus of the diaphragm.

Two important symptoms may arise from peptic esophagitis. The commoner is substernal pain; it is brought on by positions which encourage gastroesophageal reflux, mainly lying flat and stooping after a meal. The second symptom is bleeding, rarely presenting as hematemesis (vomiting of blood) but sometimes causing severe and at first obscure anemia.

DIAGNOSIS. Barium meal examination in the head-down position will establish the diagnosis as will esophagoscopy.

TREATMENT. The patient should take small, frequent meals and alkali tablets between meals. He should sleep well propped-up with pillows to prevent reflux. Surgery is also employed.

### Achalasia of the Cardia

This condition is due to degeneration of the cells of Auerbach's plexus in the lower part of the esophagus. As a result peristalsis in that region is absent and the cardia fails to relax. The esophagus becomes dilated and may contain food residues. Achalasia of the cardia may occur at any age but is more common in middle age and in women.

CLINICAL FEATURES. The chief symptoms are dysphagia and regurgitation. Radiographic examination of the esophagus in advanced cases shows it to be grossly dilated and filled with food residue. Spill-over into the lungs occurs and the patient develops recurrent attacks of pneumonia.

TREATMENT is surgical.

## Carcinoma of the Esophagus

This disease occurs much more often in men than women. The growth may occur in any part of the esophagus but more commonly the lower third. Frequently the patient can indicate fairly accurately the level at which his food appears to stick. The dysphagia is progressive so that eventually the patient has difficulty in swallowing fluids. The patient loses weight rapidly.

DIAGNOSIS. Barium swallow shows an irregular area of narrowing. Esophagoscopy enables a biopsy to be taken for histologic examination.

TREATMENT. The prognosis is extremely poor but on occasion successful surgical resection of the tumor may be possible.

# THE STOMACH AND DUODENUM

## Acute Gastritis

Acute gastritis is due to an irritant such as excessive alcohol or food poisoning or occasionally to an acute specific infection such as influenza. The symptoms are loss of appetite, nausea, vomiting and abdominal discomfort. The treatment is to avoid further irritation.

## Chronic Gastritis

The best-known variety is that due to chronic alcoholism. The patient complains of loss of appetite and nausea, particularly in the early morning, and frequently vomits mucus which has collected in the esophagus and stomach during the night. The treatment is to refrain from drinking alcohol.

## Peptic Ulcer

Peptic ulcers may be acute or chronic. They occur in the lower esophagus, stomach or duodenum and occasionally in the upper jejunum or at a gastroenterostomy stoma.

Acute ulcers cause little in the way of symptoms and are seldom diagnosed unless they cause serious bleeding or perforation. They usually heal rapidly but often recur. Aspirin is a gastric irritant and may cause superficial gastric erosions which bleed.

Nearly all chronic peptic ulcers occur in the stomach and duodenum. Both types of ulcers are more common in persons of blood group O.

Patients with duodenal ulcers secrete more acid than normal patients.

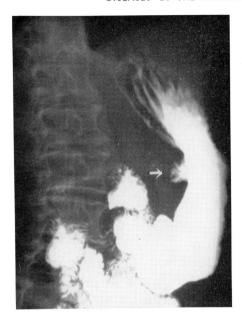

**Figure 6.1.** Gastric ulcer, lesser curvature (arrow). There is some residual food at the base of the ulcer which accounts for its irregular contour. Female, aged 40 years. (*Courtesy of Dr. Lee A. Malmed*)

Gastric ulcers, on the other hand, tend to be associated with low or normal acid secretions.

Gastric ulcers tend to occur more often than duodenal ulcers in older people. The sex incidence of gastric ulcers is almost equal; duodenal ulcers are three to four times more common in men than in women.

CLINICAL FEATURES. The principal symptom is pain which is localized to the epigastrium. It has two very characteristic features. The first is its time-relation to food: a duodenal ulcer typically causes hunger pain, which comes on when the stomach is empty and is relieved by the taking of food; with a gastric ulcer the timing is in many instances less regular but the pain tends to come on from one-half to one hour after meals. The pain of duodenal ulcer frequently wakes the patient up about 2 A.M. The patient often has a history of remissions, with complete freedom from symptoms for weeks or months. Vomiting may also occur in peptic ulceration.

DIAGNOSIS. Barium meal and radiologic screening is the most satisfactory method of diagnosis (Figures 6.1 and 6.2).

COMPLICATIONS

1. *Hemorrhage.* This may vary from slight bleeding to a massive hemorrhage. The patient may vomit a large quantity of blood. On the other hand, if the blood goes down into the intestines, large amounts of altered blood in the stools makes them black and tarry (melena).

2. *Perforation.* The discharge of acid gastric or duodenal contents into the peritoneal cavity causes an inflammatory reaction (peritonitis) with severe generalized abdominal pain and boardlike rigidity of the abdominal muscles.

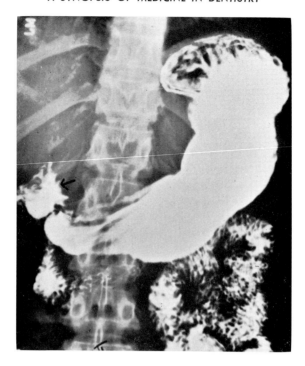

**A.**

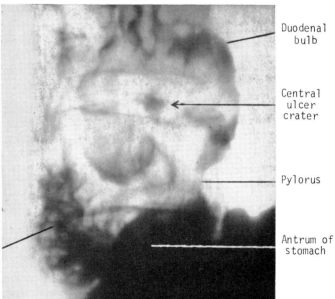

Duodenal
bulb

Central
ulcer
crater

Pylorus

Antrum of
stomach

Descending
duodenum

**B.**

**Figure 6.2.** Duodenal ulcer. **A.** A film of the upper gastrointestinal tract shows barium outlining a normal appearing stomach and a slightly deformed duodenal bulb (arrow). Male, aged 30 years. **B.** A series of compression spot film examinations of the duodenal bulb of the same patient shows a central collection of barium trapped in a duodenal ulcer (arrow). The act of compression has emptied much of the bulb to enable easier visualization of the ulcer. (*Courtesy of Dr. Lee A. Malmed*)

3. *Pyloric stenosis* is most commonly a complication of duodenal ulcer and results from contraction of scar tissue laid down in the base of the ulcer; this produces vomiting of the stomach contents.

TREATMENT OF PEPTIC ULCER

1. *Medical treatment.* Bed rest, no smoking, frequent light foods which at first consist of milk. When the pain disappears after a few days, the diet becomes more normal in character. In addition, sedatives, antacids and antispasmodics are given.

2. *Surgical treatment.* There are a number of operations available for the surgical treatment of peptic ulcer. The tendency nowadays in patients with duodenal ulcer and some patients with gastric ulcer is for the surgeon in addition to sever the vagal innervation to the stomach thus reducing gastric acid secretion and gastrin production. Recurrent ulceration is less likely following vagotomy.

## Carcinoma of the Stomach

Carcinoma of the stomach occurs slightly more often in men than women and is a common cause of death.

CLINICAL FEATURES. The condition should be suspected when a middle-aged patient develops for the first time indigestion which has been present for more than two or three weeks. The most common symptoms are anorexia and epigastric pain which usually does not show the same relationship to food as seen in patients with peptic ulcer. Later there is obvious weight loss and anemia. The patient may vomit altered blood which looks like coffee grounds.

In advanced cases, a hard mass in the epigastrium forms as well as secondary deposits in the liver.

DIAGNOSIS. This is confirmed by barium meal (Figure 6.3).

TREATMENT. Radical surgery is the only cure but the prognosis is poor.

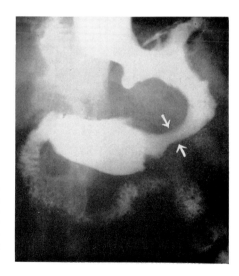

**Figure 6.3.** Carcinoma of stomach. The body of the stomach is narrowed by an infiltrating adenocarcinoma (arrows). This area was rigid at fluoroscopy, showing no peristaltic activity. Female, aged 69 years. (*Courtesy of Dr. Lee A. Malmed*)

# DISEASES OF THE INTESTINES

## Disorders of Bowel Function

Excessive peristaltic activity may on occasion be associated with pain or *colic*. This is an acute cramping pain occurring in waves or surges. The pain of small bowel colic is usually localized in the umbilicus and that of the large bowel along its general course.

Alterations in the defecation habits are referred to as diarrhea and constipation.

### Diarrhea

Diarrhea is the repeated passage of unformed stools and occurs in the following disorders:

1. *Infective conditions*
   Food poisoning
   Bacillary dysentery
   Typhoid and paratyphoid fevers
2. *Inflammatory disorders of the bowel*
   Ulcerative colitis
   Regional enteritis
   Diverticulitis
3. *Neoplasms*
   Carcinoma of the descending colon and rectum
4. *Emotional Tension*
   Irritable colon
5. *Defects of absorption*
   Malabsorption syndromes

### Constipation

Constipation is the difficult evacuation of stool because of firm consistency; it may be due to the following causes:

1. *Psychogenic causes*
   Habitual constipation or rectal dyschezia
   Irritable colon
2. *Reflex spasm of the anus*
   Anal ulcers
   Thrombosed hemorrhoids
3. *Mechanical obstruction*
   Carcinoma of the sigmoid colon
   Congenital megacolon

Insufficient bulk of material entering the colon as in starvation may result in infrequency of defecation. Defecation is a conditioned reflex and if the call to stool is persistently ignored, rectal distention ceases to evoke the desire to defecate. This is one of the most common causes of constipation and is known as rectal dyschezia. Irritable colon may give rise to constipation or diarrhea (see p. 70). Anal ulcers and hemorrhoids may cause constipation but more frequently they are the result of constipation rather than a cause.

Sigmoidoscopy and barium enema are important methods of investigating constipation of recent origin in order to exclude a carcinoma of the sigmoid colon.

In congenital megacolon there is absence of myenteric ganglion cells and absence of peristalsis in the aganglionic segment.

TREATMENT. Habitual constipation is best treated by giving meals with sufficient bulk, avoiding the use of laxatives and reestablishment of regular bowel habits. Anal lesions and mechanical obstruction require surgical treatment.

## FOOD POISONING

Certain foods such as mushrooms and shellfish when ingested occasionally may cause illness or death. In addition, food may be contaminated by salmonellae or exotoxins produced by staphylococci and rarely by *Clostridium botulinum*.

Many salmonellae serotypes commonly derived from animal sources give rise to acute food poisoning in man. Infection with these organisms is usually confined to the intestinal tract and therefore presents as gastroenteritis. After an incubation period of six to twenty-four hours the onset of the illness is sudden with fever, vomiting and diarrhea. Definitive diagnosis depends on isolation of the causative organism from the stool.

Staphylococcal enterotoxin is thermostable and is produced especially when staphylococci grow in carbohydrate foods such as pastry. Vomiting and diarrhea occur within one to six hours of ingestion of the contaminated food.

TREATMENT. The treatment is based on correction of fluid and electrolyte imbalances and not an antibiotic therapy. Antibiotics should be withheld so far as possible in infections of the alimentary tract since they may induce antibiotic resistance in normal bowel bacteria which is then transmitted to other organisms by a "resistance transfer factor." It has been shown that antibiotics, particularly chloramphenicol, prolong the carrier state and antibiotics may in themselves aggravate diarrhea.

## BACILLARY DYSENTERY

Bacillary dysentery is the result of infection of the large intestine with one of the species of *Shigella* bacilli. There are four serologic types of these nonmotile, gram-negative rods which cause bacillary dysentery in man, and these are *Shigella dysenteriae*, *Shigella flexneri*, *Shigella boydii* and *Shigella sonnei*. The disease is most common in the tropics but occurs throughout the world especially in overcrowded and unhygienic conditions. The disease is transmitted from man to man by "food, fingers, feces and flies."

6

The pathologic findings are inflammation of the wall of the colon with superficial ulceration.

CLINICAL FEATURES. After an incubation period of 48 hours there is sudden onset of abdominal pain, cramps, diarrhea and fever. The stools are liquid and contain mucus and a little blood. The disease is usually self-limiting but may lead to dehydration particularly in children.

DIAGNOSIS. Isolation of the organisms from the stool is diagnostic.

TREATMENT. Chloramphenicol or tetracycline are the preferred antibiotics. Fluid and electrolyte replacement should be given to a patient who is dehydrated.

## TYPHOID FEVER

Typhoid fever is caused by ingestion of food or drink contaminated by *Salmonella typhosa*, a gram-negative bacillus which in common with all other salmonellae fails to ferment lactose. Organisms reach the small intestine from which they enter the intestinal lymphatics and thence the bloodstream via the thoracic duct. There is hyperplasia and necrosis of the lymphoid tissue in the intestinal tract, principally Peyer's patches in the terminal ileum, leading to necrosis and ulceration. Occasionally the ulceration involves the muscular and serosal coats and intestinal perforation occurs. The liver, spleen and mesenteric lymph nodes are enlarged.

A chronic carrier state may occur after infection with *Salmonella typhosa* and is characterized by prolonged excretion of salmonellae in the feces or urine.

CLINICAL FEATURES. Classically the disease runs a course of four weeks but this has altered since the advent of antibiotic therapy. After an incubation period of eight to fourteen days the disease is ushered in with headache, general malaise, cough, abdominal tenderness and fever. These symptoms persist for about one week. During the second week the typical "rose-colored" spots appear on the chest and upper abdomen: these are two to five mm. in diameter, blanch on pressure and occur in crops. The spleen enlarges and can be palpated. The mental state may vary from confusion to delirium. Diarrhea is common during the second week and the stools may contain blood. Intestinal hemorrhage and perforation may occur during this period and death may ensue. Improvement occurs during the third and fourth weeks.

LABORATORY DIAGNOSIS. During the first week organisms can be cultured from the blood and in the second and third weeks from the stools. An increase in titer of agglutinins against the somatic (0) antigens and flagellar (H) antigens of *Salmonella typhosa* (Widal reaction) usually reaches a peak during the third week of the illness. Leukopenia is observed in many cases.

TREATMENT. Chloramphenicol is the drug of choice but ampicillin is also of value. The latter drug is used to terminate the carrier state.

PROPHYLAXIS. A course of three subcutaneous injections of 0.5 ml. of typhoid vaccine at weekly intervals is effective in the prevention of the disease. Yearly booster injections are necessary to maintain immunity.

## PARATYPHOID FEVER

Although this may be clinically indistinguishable from typhoid fever, it is usually milder with a shorter course and a lower mortality rate.

## ULCERATIVE COLITIS

This is a disease of the colon of unknown etiology although some regard it as psychosomatic in origin.

CLINICAL FEATURES. It usually starts in early adult life and is slightly more common in women than men. The patient passes large numbers of stools which contain blood and mucus. There is abdominal pain, a raised temperature, anemia and marked loss of weight.

DIAGNOSIS. The diagnosis is confirmed by sigmoidoscopy and barium enema.

COMPLICATIONS. These include stricture of the bowel, perforation and the development of carcinoma in the diseased colon.

TREATMENT. The patient should have bed rest, a high-protein diet with vitamin supplements and iron. Blood transfusion may be necessary. Cortisone is of value. In some patients, resection of the diseased bowel is carried out and a permanent ileostomy is constructed.

## REGIONAL ENTERITIS (CROHN'S DISEASE)

This is a disease of unknown etiology in which parts of the intestine, particularly the ileum, become grossly thickened by lymphoid hyperplasia, ulceration, edema and secondary infection. Complications include stenosis of the bowel, perforation, abscesses and the formation of fistulae. The sex incidence is approximately equal and symptoms usually begin in the twenties and thirties.

CLINICAL FEATURES. Most patients present with attacks of colicky pain around the umbilicus or in the right iliac fossa with associated diarrhea and general weakness. A tender fixed mass may be felt in the right iliac fossa and the barium follow-through examination will show narrowing of the affected portion of the intestine.

TREATMENT. Bed rest and sulfonamides have been used. A high-protein diet with vitamin supplements are given. Cortisone may be necessary. Surgery is employed in eliminating the complications of the disease.

## DIVERTICULITIS

Diverticula develop in the colon in about five percent of people over middle age, and the presence of diverticula is known as diverticulosis. Diverticulitis is inflammation of the diverticula.

CLINICAL FEATURES. The patient complains of colicky, lower abdominal pain associated with constipation or diarrhea. On occasion, blood is passed in the stools. Abdominal examination reveals a tender mass in relation to the affected segment of bowel.

DIAGNOSIS. Barium enema establishes the diagnosis.

TREATMENT. Most cases respond to medical treatment with antibiotics, although some patients may require surgery.

## NEOPLASMS OF THE INTESTINES

Malignant tumors of the small intestine are rare. Benign tumors do occur and may cause intussusception which is the invagination of one portion of the intestine into another. A disease of significance to the dentist is Peutz-Jeghers syndrome in which buccal and facial melanin pigmentation occurs associated with polypi of the small intestine. This disease is not precancerous as is familial polyposis coli in which polypi of the large intestine are present.

Malignant tumors of the large intestine are not uncommon. They may give rise to change in bowel habit, constipation or diarrhea, intestinal obstruction and rectal bleeding (Figure 6.4).

## IRRITABLE COLON

In this condition disturbances of colonic function accompany emotional tension. Abdominal pain is present, associated with colonic spasm. Some patients complain of constipation, others of diarrhea. Anticholinergic drugs are of value in the treatment.

## THE MALABSORPTION SYNDROMES

The malabsorption syndromes are a group of diseases which are characterized by the failure of the small intestine to absorb essential food factors

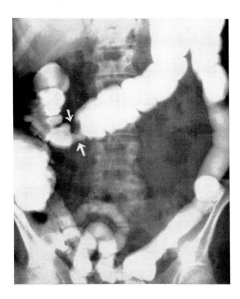

**Figure 6.4.** Carcinoma of colon. An annular, constricting lesion of the proximal transverse colon due to an infiltrating adenocarcinoma is demonstrated (arrows). Female, aged 55 years. (*Courtesy of Dr. Lee A. Malmed*)

with consequent chronic diarrhea and malnutrition. Although they are somewhat rare they are of importance to the dentist as they may be the cause of a sore tongue. The most common of the malabsorption syndromes are tropical sprue, celiac disease in children and adult celiac disease.

## Tropical Sprue

Sprue is endemic to the Far East and also the West Indies. It particularly affects Europeans who have lived for some years in those areas.

The villi undergo atrophy; it is believed that sprue results from an alteration of the normal bacterial flora of the intestines following recurrent dysenteric infection.

TREATMENT. High-protein diet and vitamin supplements are prescribed. Tetracycline 250 mg. q.i.d. for five days is also beneficial. Folic acid and vitamin $B_{12}$ are given for correction of the anemia.

## Celiac Disease

Celiac disease occurs in children between the ages of six months and six years. It is caused by intolerance to gluten. The disease is characterized by loss of appetite, failure to grow and weakness. The stools are bulky and contain excess of fat. Anemia is associated with the disorder due to folic acid or iron deficiency or both.

TREATMENT. A gluten-free diet high in calories and protein is given. Vitamin supplements are also given and the anemia is corrected.

## Adult Celiac Disease (Non-tropical Sprue)

Some adults have adult celiac disease as the continuing manifestation of the childhood disease. The patient complains of persistent diarrhea and loss of weight.

TREATMENT. This is the same as for celiac disease in children.

## Acute Appendicitis

Acute appendicitis results from an obstruction of the appendix by feces or interference with its vascular supply. It is one of the commonest acute abdominal emergencies.

CLINICAL FEATURES. The condition occurs at all ages but is less common in infants and the aged. At first, there is generalized abdominal pain which gradually becomes localized around the umbilicus. This is followed by vomiting. The right iliac fossa is tender, and pressure in the left iliac fossa accentuates the pain. The pulse and temperature are normal in the first six hours; a rise in temperature indicates complication. A leucocytosis is commonly found and is important in confirming the diagnosis.

COMPLICATIONS include perforation, gangrene, peritonitis and local abscess formation.

TREATMENT. Appendectomy and drainage of pus when present.

## Gastrointestinal Bleeding

*Hematemesis* is the vomiting of blood. In the upper gastrointestinal tract hemorrhage may occur from ruptured esophageal varices, from peptic ulceration or a gastric carcinoma. Blood may also be swallowed following a nosebleed or tooth extraction. If the blood remains in the stomach for some time before it is vomited it is altered to a dark brown color by the acid gastric juice. This distinguishes hematemesis from hemoptysis which is the expectoration of bright red, frothy blood from the respiratory tract.

Instead of being vomited the blood may pass down the gastrointestinal tract to be voided in the stools. Small amounts of blood do not discolor the feces and this is known as *occult bleeding*. If the bleeding continues over a long enough period of time an iron deficiency anemia may ensue (p. 92).

Melena is the passage of black, tarry stools resulting from hemorrhage usually proximal to the ileocecal valve.

The passage of bright red blood in the stools is usually the result of bleeding from the lower bowel. The common causes are hemorrhoids, diverticulitis, ulcerative colitis and carcinoma.

## Intestinal Obstruction (Ileus)

Obstruction of the intestinal contents may result from mechanical blockage of the lumen or by paralysis of the bowel wall (paralytic ileus). If the obstruction is complete then death will ensue unless the obstruction is relieved. Tumors of the bowel, fibrous bands and interference with the blood supply to the intestine are common causes of mechanical obstruction. Obstructions with strangulation (impairment of the blood supply leading to necrosis of tissue) occur in hernias and as a result of volvulus (twisting) or intussusception. Infarction or necrosis of the bowel wall occurs unless the blood supply is quickly restored.

Paralytic ileus most commonly ensues after operation or as a result of peritonitis.

Obstruction may occur in the small or large bowel. In the small bowel, obstruction causes excessive vomiting with dehydration and electrolyte disturbances. In low intestinal obstruction, dehydration and electrolyte loss are not as frequent and the cause of death is thought to be due to absorption of toxic material from the injured intestinal wall.

In complete intestinal obstruction neither feces nor flatus (gas) are passed.

CLINICAL FEATURES. In small bowel obstruction recurring attacks of severe abdominal pain occur localized mainly at the umbilicus. Copious vomiting occurs. Visible peristalsis may be present. In paralytic ileus, pain is frequently absent but the patient may complain of abdominal discomfort. Normal bowel sounds which accompany peristalsis are lost in paralytic ileus.

In large bowel obstruction there is a history of increasing constipation that finally becomes absolute (obstipation). Colicky pains are experienced along the course of the large bowel and the cecum becomes ballooned.

A plain radiograph of the abdomen will show when the jejunum, ileum or the colon is distended with gas; each has a characteristic appearance that allows it to be distinguished radiologically.

In large bowel obstructions sigmoidoscopy and barium enema are employed in the evaluation of the patient.

TREATMENT. This is three-fold: (1) gastrointestinal suction; (2) replacement and maintenance of fluid and electrolyte balance; (3) relief of the obstruction by operation.

## DISEASES OF THE LIVER, GALLBLADDER AND BILE DUCTS

The liver, which is the largest organ in the body, possesses great regenerative powers and has many functions. These include the formation of bile, urea, serum albumin, fibrinogen, prothrombin, heparin, glycogen and ketones. In addition, the detoxification of toxins, deamination of proteins, storage of glycogen and excretion of drugs also occur in the liver.

### Diagnostic Tests

#### LIVER FUNCTION TESTS

The purpose of liver function tests is to ascertain whether the liver is functioning normally as well as to distinguish between the different types of jaundice. Hepatic disease is often characterized by alterations in plasma protein fractions which may be detected by electrophoresis.

#### Serum Albumin

The normal serum albumin level is 3.5 to 5.5 Gm. per 100 ml. of serum. In chronic liver disease cellular damage is associated with a lowering of the serum albumin and edema results.

#### Prothrombin Time

The one-stage prothrombin time of Quick is useful in differentiating deficiencies caused by abnormal vitamin K absorption from those due to liver-cell dysfunction. Biliary obstruction interferes with absorption of this vitamin; when it is administered parenterally, the prothrombin returns to normal. In contrast, in jaundice and hypothrombinemia due to liver-cell damage, vitamin K has little or no effect on the prothrombin time.

#### Dye Excretion by the Liver

Bromsulphthalein (BSP) is injected intravenously to assess the functional state of the liver. Normally three percent to five percent remains in the serum 45 minutes following administration. Elevation of the amount of BSP 45 minutes after administration indicates hepatocellular damage. The BSP test is of greater value in the absence of jaundice.

## Flocculation Tests

The thymol turbidity and the cephalin cholesterol flocculation tests are empirical tests which are useful in confirming the presence of hepatocellular damage.

## Serum Alkaline Phosphatase

The alkaline phosphatase level is elevated in obstructive jaundice.

## Serum Transaminases

The enzymes serum glutamic-oxaloacetic (GOT) and glutamic-pyruvic (GPT) transaminases are raised in liver damage and also in myocardial infarction. Normal serum contains $<40$ Karmen units of GOT and $<30$ Karmen units of GPT.

## PHOTOSCANS OF THE LIVER

Gamma-emitting radioisotopes such as $I^{131}$ rose bengal and $Au^{198}$ are used in the diagnosis of metastatic malignancy in the liver, hepatic abscess and parasitic and other cysts. $I^{131}$ rose bengal is largely concentrated in the parenchymal hepatic cells, whereas $Au^{198}$ is taken up in the Kupffer cells.

## LIVER BIOPSY

Liver biopsy is used to make or to confirm a diagnosis of liver disease. It is not employed in patients with a prolonged prothrombin time.

## Diseases of the Liver

## JAUNDICE

Jaundice is the yellow discoloration of the tissues with bile pigment. The skin, oral mucosa and sclerotics are colored yellow; the color may vary from a light yellow to a deep greenish-yellow.

## Physiology of Bile

The hemoglobin derived from the breakdown of red corpuscles in the reticuloendothelial system is split into two parts: an iron-containing part which is resynthesized in the bone marrow to hemoglobin and an iron-free porphyrin fraction. From the latter, bilirubin is derived. When passed into the bloodstream, the bilirubin is insoluble in water; it is, therefore, unable to pass into the urine and gives an indirect van den Bergh reaction. After passage through the liver, bilirubin is modified to give a direct van den Bergh reaction. This modified bilirubin passes down the bile ducts to the intestine where it is converted to stercobilinogen which is the pigment responsible for the normal color of the feces. Some of this is absorbed as urobilinogen from the small intestine and small amounts are excreted in the urine.

## Hemolytic Jaundice

There are three main varieties of jaundice. In hemolytic jaundice there is abnormally rapid breakdown of the red cells in the circulation leading to an increase in the level of bilirubin in the serum. The liver is unable to dispose of the large amounts of insoluble bilirubin formed and the latter passes into the intestine where it is converted into stercobilinogen. An excess of urobilinogen is excreted in the urine but the stools are normal in color. Hemolytic jaundice is the least common form.

## Obstructive Jaundice

In this form of jaundice obstruction of the common bile duct occurs. Consequently, no bile passes into the intestine and the stools are pale. The patient often complains of pruritus and bradycardia is associated with the disorder. The most frequent causes of occlusion of the common bile duct are gallstones and carcinoma of the head of the pancreas or of the ampulla of Vater. In this type of jaundice, the serum alkaline phosphatase level is raised but it is never as high as in Paget's disease.

## Hepatic Jaundice

The liver cells are damaged in this type of jaundice. The findings are similar to obstructive jaundice except that the liver function tests show evidence of liver damage.

## Tooth Extraction in Jaundiced Patients

Before tooth extraction the prothrombin time is ascertained. If this is increased, vitamin $K_1$ is given orally or intramuscularly in doses of five to twenty mg.

## CIRRHOSIS OF THE LIVER

In cirrhosis of the liver there is necrosis of liver cells which results in loss of normal architecture of the liver lobules associated with an increase of fibrous tissue. In addition, regeneration of parenchymal cells occurs.

The three commonest forms of cirrhosis are fatty nutritional cirrhosis (Laennec's cirrhosis), biliary cirrhosis and postnecrotic cirrhosis.

## Fatty Nutritional Cirrhosis (Laennec's Cirrhosis, Portal Cirrhosis)

This disorder is believed to be related to nutritional disturbances which induce fatty changes in the liver followed by the development of cirrhosis. In the United States the most common cause of this disease is chronic alcoholism but in the underdeveloped countries protein deficiency (kwashiorkor) has been implicated. Cirrhosis following chronic alcoholism is more common in males than females and occurs principally in the age group between 40 and 60 years. Protein deficiency and cirrhosis due to this cause are seen more frequently in children.

Varices at the lower end of the esophagus develop in cirrhosis of the liver because of obstruction of the portal circulation. Hemorrhage from the varices results from increased hydrostatic pressure and mucosal ulceration.

CLINICAL FEATURES. In some patients the disease may present insidiously with anorexia, fatigue and weakness followed by a gradual onset of jaundice and ascites. In others there may be acute upper gastrointestinal bleeding (from ruptured esophageal varices), sudden onset of ascites (excess fluid in the peritoneal cavity), and liver failure with jaundice or coma. Examination of the patient will reveal a firm, enlarged, nontender liver with or without an enlarged spleen, spider angiomas and the typical erythema of the palms.

TREATMENT. In cirrhosis due to chronic alcoholism, the patient should stop drinking alcohol. An adequate diet is given containing proteins, vitamins and minerals. When anemia is present, iron is administered. In patients with ascites, salt is restricted. When the patient presents with gastrointestinal bleeding, blood transfusion is given and measures are taken to stop the bleeding. Hepatic coma is treated by restriction of dietary protein, by enemas to remove nitrogenous bowel contents and by neomycin to reduce the bacterial flora.

## Biliary Cirrhosis

Primary biliary cirrhosis is of unknown etiology although some authorities believe that there may be an autoimmune basis. In secondary biliary cirrhosis the typical histopathologic changes of cirrhosis occur secondary to bile duct obstruction with or without infection.

CLINICAL FEATURES. Primary biliary cirrhosis occurs most commonly in women aged 40 to 60 in whom the earliest symptom may be generalized pruritus. Early in the disease the liver is usually enlarged and firm and the spleen is palpable. Later, jaundice with dark urine and pale stools and xanthomas of the skin are seen. As stasis increases within the biliary tree the manifestations of malabsorption may become evident: weight loss, diarrhea with pale bulky stools, bleeding due to hypoprothrombinemia and collapse of vertebrae, and pathologic fractures with bone demineralization due to malabsorption of vitamin D and calcium.

TREATMENT. Supplements of vitamin $K_1$ (five to ten mg.) and vitamins A and D (10,000 units) are given by mouth daily with calcium lactate or gluconate, six to twelve grams. Pruritus may be relieved with methyl testosterone.

DENTAL IMPLICATIONS. See under tooth extraction in jaundiced patients (p. 79).

## Postnecrotic Cirrhosis

Postnecrotic cirrhosis may follow acute viral hepatitis or may be idiopathic in origin. The liver in this condition is typically reduced in size.

CLINICAL FEATURES. Late in the disease spider angiomata of the skin are seen together with splenic enlargement. Ascites, hepatic coma and bleeding from esophageal varices are found.

TREATMENT. The treatment is as for fatty nutritional cirrhosis.

## Disorders of the Gallbladder

### GALLSTONES

Gallstones are composed of cholesterol, calcium bilirubinate and calcium carbonate. About 10 percent of gallstones are composed entirely of one of these constituents. Mixed gallstones are the commonest variety. Important factors in the formation of gallstones are disturbances of cholesterol metabolism, infection and stasis (Figure 6.5).

### ACUTE CHOLECYSTITIS

This condition is commonly associated with obstruction of the cystic duct by a stone; the wall of the gallbladder is inflamed as a result of chemical damage by concentrated bile. Bacterial infection, produced by bacteria in the gastrointestinal tract, may be superimposed and in some cases pus may fill the gallbladder (empyema).

CLINICAL FEATURES. The onset is sudden and the patient complains of agonizing pain in the right upper quadrant of the abdomen below the ribs. Severe nausea and vomiting occur. Usually the temperature is raised to 101° F or more. On the second or third day of the attack there may be slight jaundice. Palpation of the abdomen reveals tenderness and rigidity in the right upper quadrant and sometimes the enlarged gallbladder can be felt.

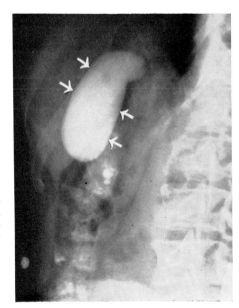

**Figure 6.5.** Gallstones. Gallbladder contrast material administered orally 16 hours earlier is well concentrated within the gallbladder. Note the presence of four radiolucent defects representing gallstones (arrows). Some contrast material is seen in the adjacent intestine. Male, aged 61 years. (*Courtesy of Dr. Lee A. Malmed*)

TREATMENT. Some authorities favor conservative treatment of continuous gastric aspiration, intravenous dextrose saline solution, meperidine for pain, propantheline bromide (probanthine) to reduce gastric and pancreatic secretion and relieve spasm and tetracyclines to control infection. When the acute symptoms have subsided cholecystectomy (removal of the gallbladder) is carried out. Other authorities favor immediate cholecystotomy (drainage of the gallbladder) followed by cholecystectomy at a later date.

## DISEASES OF THE PANCREAS

### Acute Pancreatitis

Acute pancreatitis is believed to be brought about by increased pancreatic secretion with partial or complete obstruction of outflow and raised intraductal pressure. The increased intraductal pressure results in rupture of the ducts and release of enzymes into the tissues. The enzymes act upon blood vessels and parenchyma, producing hemorrhage and necrosis. Areas of fat necrosis occur in the pancreas, mesentery and omentum. The condition may be precipitated by a heavy meal or by alcohol both of which cause increased pancreatic secretion. It may also occur following a heavy blow on the abdomen or following surgery in the upper abdomen.

CLINICAL FEATURES. The disease affects adults of any age and is more common in men than in women. The patient complains of severe pain in the upper abdomen which radiates to the back, chest and lower abdomen. Nausea and vomiting, abdominal distention and constipation occur frequently. Mild jaundice usually follows within one to three days of the onset. The condition of the patient may vary from distressed and anxious to severe shock. Tenderness and spasm in the upper abdomen are present.

Acute pancreatitis is accompanied by leucocytosis, increased serum amylase in the early stages to values exceeding 250 Somogyi units, increased serum lipase and increased amylase in the urine. One quarter of the patients have glucosuria.

TREATMENT. Shock is treated with plasma, human albumin and electrolyte solutions. Continuous gastric suction is employed for several days to reduce intestinal secretions, meperidine is given to control pain, and propantheline bromide is administered to inhibit pancreatic secretion.

### Cystic Fibrosis (Fibrocystic Disease, Mucoviscidosis)

Cystic fibrosis is a hereditary disease which is transmitted by a recessive gene. The patient is a homozygote and his healthy parents heterozygote. The disease affects both mucus-secreting and nonmucus-secreting exocrine glands and there is increased viscosity of mucus and a high sodium chloride content of sweat. The increased sodium and chloride of sweat is used as a diagnostic test. Within the bronchial lumen, thick, tenacious secretions are found which lead to bronchial obstruction and secondary infection resulting finally in bronchiectasis. There is a tendency for staphylococcal bronchopneumonia to develop and chronic sinus infection is common. The pancreatic enzyme is deficient.

CLINICAL FEATURES. These are cough associated with the production of large quantities of mucopurulent sputum, hemoptysis and recurrent pneumonia. The fingers and toes are often clubbed. The breath is frequently foul-smelling. Moist rales are heard over the affected areas of the lungs.

Despite a huge appetite the patient fails to thrive, has frequent large foul stools and a protuberant abdomen.

TREATMENT. A high-protein, high-caloric diet is given with vitamin supplement. The missing pancreatic enzymes are replaced by pancreatin powder. Additional salt and fluid are given in hot weather to replace the sweat loss.

Drainage of the bronchi is effected by postural drainage, breathing exercises and physical activity. If the patient has a raised temperature and increase in the quantity of mucopurulent sputum, a course of antibiotic therapy is given based on the sensitivity of the organisms.

## GENERAL REFERENCES

Beeson, P. B. and McDermott, W.: *Cecil-Loeb Textbook of Medicine*, 13th ed., Philadelphia, Saunders, 1971.

Harrison, T. R., Adams, R. D., Bennett, I. L., Resnik, W. H., Thorn, G. W., and Wintrobe, M. M.: *Principles of Internal Medicine*, 5th ed., New York, McGraw-Hill, 1966.

Jawetz, E., Melnick, J. L., and Adelberg, E. A.: *Review of Medical Microbiology*, 8th ed., Los Altos, Lange, 1968.

Moyer, C. A., Rhoads, J. E., Allen, J. G., and Harkins, H. N.: *Surgery, Principles and Practice*, 3rd ed., Philadelphia, Lippincott, 1965.

Ramsay, A. M.: Acute infective diarrhea. Brit. Med. J., *2*, 347, 1968.

# DISEASES OF THE BLOOD

The blood contains three cellular elements: erythrocytes (red cells), leucocytes (white cells) and thrombocytes (platelets). Each has its own function and life span. In health, destruction is balanced by production and the levels of circulating cells remain remarkably constant. Within the bone marrow are formed the red cells, granulocytes and platelets. The lymphocytes and monocytes are formed in the lymphoid tissue throughout the body including the bone marrow.

## Plasma Proteins

The plasma proteins include fibrinogen, albumin and globulin and constitute 6–8 Gms./100 ml. of the plasma. With the exception of $\gamma$-globulins, the plasma proteins are formed in the liver. Fibrinogen is important in the clotting mechanism. Albumin and globulin exert an osmotic pressure which opposes the hydrostatic pressure in the capillaries. The globulin fraction comprises alpha-1, alpha-2, beta and gamma components. The approximate concentrations in human plasma can be determined by electrophoretic analysis.

## Immunoglobulins

The immunoglobulins (antibodies) are produced by the plasma cells. Each immunoglobulin consists of four polypeptide chains, two heavy polypeptide chains and two light chains, linked by disulfide bonds. The light chains, which are common to all of the major classes, are of two types, designated kappa ($\kappa$) and lambda ($\lambda$). The heavy chains are specific for

84

each class and have been designated gamma ($\gamma$) for IgG, alpha ($\alpha$) for IgA, mu ($\mu$) for IgM, delta ($\delta$) for IgD and epsilon ($\epsilon$) for IgE, the five major classes of human immunoglobulins. Most of the antibodies to viruses, toxins and gram-positive pyogenic bacteria are in the IgG fraction.

There are a number of pathologic conditions associated with quantitative alterations in the immunoglobulins. A deficiency of gamma globulins is found in the rare disease, agammaglobulinemia. Individuals with this condition are unable to synthesize gamma globulins and are susceptible to infectious diseases.

An increase in IgM or macroglobulins in the blood is termed macroglobulinemia and may occur as a secondary phenomenon in neoplastic diseases, collagen disorders, chronic infections, amyloidosis and hepatic cirrhosis. In the primary macroglobulinemia of Waldenström, oral ulceration and hemorrhages occur together with slight to moderate lymphadenopathy and hepatosplenomegaly.

In multiple myeloma, a neoplasm of plasma cells, Bence Jones protein is found in plasma and urine. Bence Jones protein typically precipitates upon heating to 50° to 60° C and redissolves with more heating. The disease is characterized by multiple "punched out" lesions of the bone observed on radiographic examination.

## CONDITIONS AFFECTING THE RED BLOOD CELLS

The non-nucleated red cells in the peripheral blood are derived from nucleated precursors in the bone narrow. Normoblastic erythropoiesis signifies normal morphology of the nucleated erythrocytic precursors; megaloblastic erythropoiesis indicates the abnormal morphology of erythrocytic elements which occurs in vitamin $B_{12}$ or folic acid deficiency.

A number of substances are necessary for the production of normal red blood cells. Large amounts of hemoglobin must be synthesized and this necessitates a plentiful supply of protein and iron. In addition, for normal erythropoiesis vitamin $B_{12}$, folic acid, vitamin $B_6$ and ascorbic acid are required. Traces of copper and cobalt have been shown to be essential for erythropoiesis in animals. Certain hormones play a role in maintaining red cell production since, in their absence, anemia may develop. Adrenal glucocorticoids, thyroid hormones and androgens are stimulants of red cell production. Pituitary hormones may also play a role in red cell formation mediated through the adrenal and thyroid glands and the gonads.

Erythropoietin produced by the kidney stimulates erythrocyte production (p. 57).

IRON METABOLISM. Iron is absorbed mainly in the duodenum as the bivalent (ferrous) form. Ascorbic acid appears to facilitate the absorption both by chelation of iron and by promoting reduction of the ferric to the ferrous form. Achlorhydria is associated with diminished iron absorption, since an acid pH is needed to solubilize ferric ion for chelation with ascorbic acid and other substances, in which form it is absorbed. The absorbed iron is then bound to transferrin, a $\beta_1$ globulin, and transported to the bone marrow for hemoglobin synthesis. The normal serum iron-binding capacity is around 300 $\mu$g./100 ml. (the range is 250 to 400) and is about one third saturated. The iron-binding capacity is decreased in the presence of acute or chronic infections and in the nephrotic syndrome; it is increased in iron deficiency anemia, acute hepatitis and the last trimester of pregnancy. The normal serum iron is about 100 $\mu$g./100 ml. (range 75 to 175) and is firmly chelated with transferrin. Iron requirements are increased in childhood during growth periods, in pregnancy and lactation.

IRON STORAGE. In the normal adult the iron stores amount to about 1.0 to 1.5 Gm. Most of this iron is in the liver, spleen and bone marrow and is about equally divided between ferritin and hemosiderin and is available for hemoglobin synthesis.

## Definitions

Anemia is a decrease in the level of hemoglobin below the level previously established as normal with respect to age and sex. An increase above normal with respect to age and sex in the erythrocyte count, the hemoglobin level and hematocrit is termed polycythemia.

## Anemia

Anemia may be caused by blood loss either as a result of hemorrhage or hemolysis or by impaired blood formation. There are a number of different types of anemia resulting from impaired blood formation the most important of which are due to deficiencies of vitamin $B_{12}$, folic acid and iron. Defective hemoglobin synthesis occurs in the hereditary hemoglobinopathies and results in anemia. It should be remembered that the bone marrow may be encroached upon by leukemic tissue in lymphocytic leukemia and by carcinomatous tissue in metastatic carcinoma and that in both these diseases anemia is associated. In chronic infections and liver disease there may be an associated anemia the etiology of which is unknown.

## Morphologic Classification of Anemia

Depending on the size of the erythrocyte an anemia is categorized as normocytic, microcytic or macrocytic. Red cells which have a normal concentration of hemoglobin are described as normochromic, regardless of their size. If the concentration falls below normal, the cells are termed hypochromic. The term hyperchromic does not exist with respect to mammalian erythrocytes which cannot become supersaturated with hemoglobin. Thus an anemia is categorized as normochromic or hypochromic. Most anemias are normocytic-normochromic, microcytic-hypochromic or macrocytic-normochromic (megaloblastic anemias).

In the newborn the hemoglobin varies between 18 and 22 Gm./100 ml. of blood—normal childhood levels being reached by the third month. During the first two years of life the average hemoglobin is about 11 Gm./100

TABLE 7.1. NORMAL RANGE OF BLOOD CELL VALUES

| | Men | Women | Children—both sexes (3 mo.–13 yr.) |
|---|---|---|---|
| Erythrocytes (millions/cu.mm.) | 4.6–6.2 | 4.2–5.4 | 3.8–5.2 |
| Hemoglobin (Gm./100 ml.) | 14.0–18.0 | 12.0–16.0 | 10.0–14.5 |
| Hematocrit (%) | 42–52 | 37–47 | 31–43 |

ml.; the hemoglobin and hematocrit levels and the erythrocyte count then increase slowly throughout childhood and reach adult levels at about the age of 14.

The mean corpuscular volume (MCV) and the mean corpuscular hemoglobin concentration (MCHC) are measurements which are used in the laboratory diagnosis of anemia. These values are based on averages and are inaccurate. For this reason an anemia is best classified morphologically by the examination of a well-stained blood film by a trained observer.

### Reticulocyte Count

This test serves to determine the rate of red cell production in the bone marrow. Normally between 0.5 and 2.5 percent of the red cells are reticulocytes and can be stained with stains such as brilliant cresyl blue when the basophilic material within the cell is precipitated into a reticular pattern. When the bone marrow cells are very active (a situation which occurs after hemorrhage and with recovery from anemia) there is an increase in the number of reticulocytes in the blood.

### General Aspects of Anemia

A reduction in the hemoglobin level of the blood results in tissue hypoxia. The physiologic adjustments which occur include tachycardia, an increased cardiac output, an increase in the velocity of blood flow and increased pulmonary ventilation. The release of oxygen to the tissues is improved because of the tissue hypoxia and a shift to the right of the oxyhemoglobin dissociation curve. Other manifestations of anemia include headache, low grade fever, cardiac murmurs and changes in the electrocardiogram.

The time taken for physiologic changes to occur is dependent on the rate at which the anemia develops. If a patient loses rapidly one third (or even less) of the blood volume shock will develop (p. 43).

When the anemia develops gradually as a result of chronic hemorrhage an otherwise normal person may tolerate as much as 50 percent reduction in hemoglobin without untoward effects. In patients with underlying cardiac disease or coronary insufficiency a moderate degree of anemia may precipitate congestive failure or contribute to myocardial ischemia.

7

## NORMOCYTIC-NORMOCHROMIC ANEMIAS

This group of anemias is caused by acute blood loss, by hemolysis or by decreased blood formation in the bone marrow. The red cells are normal in volume and in hemoglobin concentration. The bone marrow responds by increased erythrocyte production and as a result in the peripheral blood nucleated red cells are found along with an increase in the number of reticulocytes.

### Hemolytic Anemias

In the hemolytic anemias, the life span of the red cell is diminished. Because of the increased hemoglobin breakdown, the amount of urinary and fecal urobilinogen is increased. An increased reticulocyte count is found.

The hemolytic anemias can be conveniently divided into:

1. *Congenital*
   a. Congenital spherocytosis—no abnormal hemoglobin electrophoretic pattern
   b. Hemoglobinopathies—the hemoglobin electrophoretic pattern is abnormal
   c. Congenital deficiency of glucose-6-phosphate dehydrogenase
2. *Acquired*—due to infections and drugs

**CONGENITAL SPHEROCYTOSIS.** Patients with this condition have spherical erythrocytes which contain a normal amount of hemoglobin and which, because of their shape, are easily trapped and destroyed by the spleen.

CLINICAL FEATURES. As a rule, the patient is pale and slightly jaundiced. Because of the increased breakdown of erythrocytes, the patient tends to develop gallstones mainly of bilirubin. The spleen is enlarged, and some patients develop chronic leg ulcers.

LABORATORY FINDINGS will reveal anemia and spherocytosis. The erythrocytes show increased fragility which can be demonstrated by the osmotic fragility test.

TREATMENT. Splenectomy.

**HEMOGLOBINOPATHIES.** The hemoglobinopathies include sickle cell trait, sickle cell anemia and thalassemia minor and major.

In the blood of a normal adult, three different types of hemoglobin can be recognized:

1. Adult hemoglobin, A
2. Fetal hemoglobin, F
3. Hemoglobin $A_2$

Adult hemoglobin comprises about 97 percent hemoglobin A, about 1 percent hemoglobin F and approximately 2 percent hemoglobin $A_2$. In the newborn infant, the amount of hemoglobin F is about 80 percent and in the first year of life, this is replaced by hemoglobin A. In the United States, the most important hemoglobinopathies are hemoglobin S disease and thalassemia.

*Hemoglobin S Disease.* Hemoglobin S differs from hemoglobin A by virtue of the substitution of a single amino acid, valine, for glutamic acid in the globin portion of the molecule. Two forms of hemoglobin S disease are encountered, the heterozygous state (sickle cell trait) and the homozygous state (sickle cell anemia).

HETEROZYGOUS STATE (SICKLE CELL TRAIT). The sickle cell trait is carried by approximately 8 percent of the Negroes in the United States. Hemoglobin electrophoresis shows that 35 percent to 45 percent of the hemoglobin A is replaced by hemoglobin S. Sickling of the red cells is observed when blood is sealed under a cover slip at a low oxygen tension (Figure 7.1).

CLINICAL FEATURES. The patients are usually asymptomatic under normal conditions. However, should these individuals be exposed to a low oxygen tension, such as during anesthesia, intravascular sickling occurs. This may result in infarcts usually in the spleen and bones.

HOMOZYGOUS STATE (SICKLE CELL ANEMIA). Sickle cell anemia occurs in about one percent of American Negroes. Hemoglobin electrophoresis reveals complete absence of hemoglobin A and an increase of hemoglobin F up to 20 percent.

CLINICAL FEATURES. Patients with this form of hemoglobin S disease are

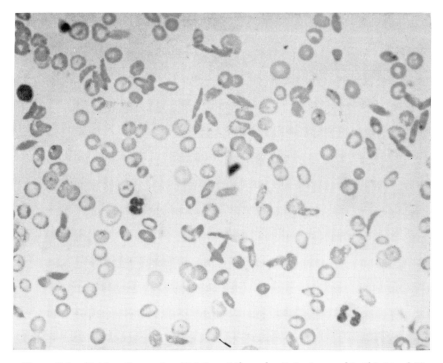

**Figure 7.1.** Sickle cell anemia. Sickling of the red cells is observed in this blood film sealed under a cover slip at low oxygen tension.

usually tall and thin and do not live much past the age of 30 years. They become adapted to the degree of anemia but frequently experience episodes of aching pains in the bones and joints and in the abdomen. The patients are pale and frequently jaundiced and the liver is enlarged. In infancy, the spleen is enlarged but diminishes in size as splenic infarcts are replaced by fibrous tissue.

Blood examination shows a marked anemia with conspicuous variation in shape of the erythrocytes. Some of the latter may also show the typical elongated appearance. Reticulocytes are found in increased numbers and nucleated red cells occur in the blood film. Death usually results from heart failure, infections or thromboses in vital organs.

ROENTGENOGRAPHIC FEATURES. Bony trabeculations are seen radiating from the skull producing a "hair-on-end" appearance. The medullary spaces of the jaw bones are frequently enlarged (Figure 7.2).

TREATMENT. Blood transfusions are given. Pain is treated with analgesics and opiates.

*Thalassemia* arises probably as a result of impairment of hemoglobin synthesis. The incidence of the condition is high in individuals of Mediterranean extraction and in Thailand. It occurs as both the heterozygous and homozygous states.

HETEROZYGOUS STATE (THALASSEMIA MINOR). Affected patients may be asymptomatic or may present with mild fatigue, jaundice,

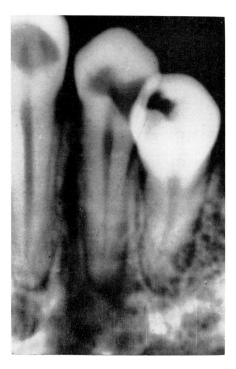

**Figure 7.2.** Sickle cell anemia. Note the enlarged medullary spaces in this periapical radiograph of the mandibular premolar teeth.

splenomegaly and anemia. The hemoglobin concentration is always below normal. Changes in the morphology of the red cells include hypochromia, microcytosis, poikilocytosis and targeting. The target cell characteristically has a densely staining center and periphery with a pale zone between the two.

HOMOZYGOUS STATE (THALASSEMIA MAJOR, COOLEY'S DISEASE). The condition first manifests in infancy or early childhood and is characterized by stunted growth, pallor, slight jaundice and marked enlargement of the liver and spleen. Typically, the child has a large head with a high forehead, the eyes are set wide apart and epicanthal folds are frequently present. In later life, the patient develops enlargement of the heart and signs of congestive cardiac failure. The anemia is always severe with a low hemoglobin concentration. Similar blood changes are found as in thalassemia minor and, in addition, nucleated red cells are found in the peripheral blood. Patients with thalassemia major rarely survive beyond the age of 20 to 25 years.

ROENTGENOGRAPHIC FEATURES. The entire skeleton shows various degrees of osteoporosis. In the skull, there is thickening of the diploë, loss of definition of the inner and outer tables and the formation of new bony trabeculae at right angles to the surface of the skull, producing a "hair-on-end" effect similar to that seen in sickle cell anemia.

TREATMENT. Blood transfusions are needed to correct the anemia.

**GLUCOSE-6-PHOSPHATE DEHYDROGENASE DEFICIENCY.** Approximately 13 percent of American Negro males and some males of Mediterranean ethnic groups will, on ingestion of certain chemicals, drugs or fava beans, develop a hemolytic anemia. The cause is related to a deficiency of glucose-6-phosphate dehydrogenase in the erythrocyte and is sex-linked. One of the drugs which commonly produces hemolysis is an antimalarial, primaquine.

**ACQUIRED HEMOLYTIC ANEMIAS.** Exposure to a number of chemical agents may produce hemolysis. Some will produce symptoms only in susceptible individuals (as in primaquine sensitivity) while others will produce symptoms in any individual if given in large enough doses. Of the latter group arsenic, lead, benzene, phenacetin and acetanilid are the most important.

**AUTOIMMUNE HEMOLYTIC ANEMIAS.** This group of hemolytic anemias is caused by the production of antibodies that destroy the patient's own red cells. They may be idiopathic or secondary to an underlying pathologic process.

The antibodies involved can be differentiated into two groups—"warm" and "cold"—according to the temperature at which they exert their maximum effect. Both types of antibody are frequently "incomplete"; that is, they do not cause agglutination when the red cells are suspended in saline. Incomplete antibodies adherent to the surface of the red cells can be detected by the use of antihuman gamma globulin (Coombs' test).

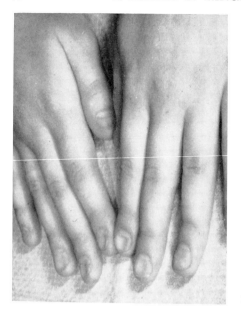

**Figure 7.3.** Koilonychia. There is extreme spooning of the nails of this female patient, aged 30 years, with severe iron-deficiency anemia.

## MICROCYTIC-HYPOCHROMIC ANEMIA (IRON DEFICIENCY ANEMIA)

This type of anemia is due to excessive loss of iron as a result of chronic hemorrhage from hemorrhoids, peptic ulcer or heavy menstrual flow or from deficient intake of iron in the diet. It may also be idiopathic.

CLINICAL FEATURES. The patient complains of weakness, breathlessness and loss of appetite. The skin is pale and the nails are spoon-shaped (koilonychia) (Figure 7.3). Cracks may occur at the angles of the mouth (angular cheilitis) and the tongue may be smooth and atrophic. The patient may complain of difficulty in swallowing and this type of dysphagia is known as the Plummer-Vinson syndrome. There is a significant increase in postcricoid carcinoma in patients with this syndrome. The plasma iron falls below 50 $\mu$g./100 ml. and plasma iron-binding capacity increases. The red cells are small and hypochromic. The hemoglobin and hematocrit levels are lower than normal.

TREATMENT. Oral iron is administered. Occasionally the anemia is unresponsive to oral iron therapy and parenteral iron is required.

## MACROCYTIC-NORMOCHROMIC ANEMIAS (MEGALOBLASTIC ANEMIAS)

In this group of anemias, there is an abnormal (megaloblastic) maturation of the red cells. Vitamin $B_{12}$ and folic acid are necessary for the full maturation of the red cell and the intrinsic factor secreted by the stomach is necessary for the absorption of vitamin $B_{12}$. In the megaloblastic anemias, the cells are reduced in number and contain the normal amount of hemoglobin. This group includes pernicious anemia and some anemias due to defective absorption of vitamin $B_{12}$ and folic acid from the small intestine. Classic examples of folic acid deficiency are tropical sprue and celiac disease (p. 75). In the latter diseases, there is diarrhea associated with sore tongue.

## Pernicious Anemia

Pernicious anemia is due to absence or deficiency of intrinsic factor which results in a deficient supply of vitamin $B_{12}$ to the bone marrow.

CLINICAL FEATURES. The patient has the usual symptoms of anemia, i.e. dyspnea, lassitude, headaches and palpitations in addition to a lemon-yellow tint to the skin in severe cases and a red, smooth and painful tongue devoid of papillae. Subacute combined degeneration of the spinal cord occurs giving rise to numbness and tingling in the feet and hands with weakness and unsteadiness in walking. Examination of the blood reveals red cells which vary in size and shape and the leukocyte count is low (Figure 7.4). Giant epithelial cells are found in exfoliative cytologic smears from the oral cavity. Characteristically, the stomach is unable to secrete free hydrochloric acid even after maximal stimulation with histamine. The serum vitamin $B_{12}$ is reduced (normal 200 to 800 $\mu\mu$g./ml.).

THE SCHILLING TEST. This test which is a urinary excretion technique is used to measure the absorption of radioactive vitamin $B_{12}$; the vitamin is

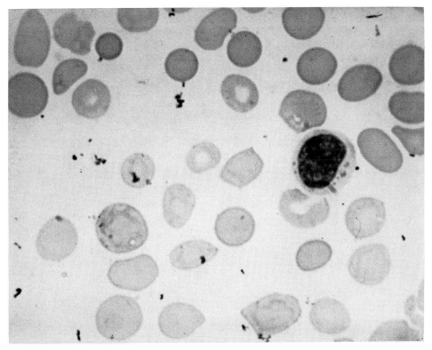

**Figure 7.4.** Pernicious anemia. Blood-film showing variation in size and shape of the red cells.

labelled with $Co^{57}$ which has a half-life of 270 days. When a small amount of radioactive vitamin $B_{12}$ is given orally and followed within one to three hours by a "flushing" dose of 1.0 mg. of nonradioactive vitamin $B_{12}$ given intramuscularly, normal subjects excrete in their urine during the following 24 hours more than 15 percent of the administered radioactivity. Individuals with impaired absorption of vitamin $B_{12}$ excrete less than five percent (most patients with pernicious anemia excrete less than two percent). In patients with impaired absorption of vitamin $B_{12}$ due to inadequate intrinsic factor production the urinary radioactivity will increase fivefold if intrinsic factor is given together with the radioactive vitamin $B_{12}$.

TREATMENT. Vitamin $B_{12}$ by injection.

## APLASTIC ANEMIA

Aplastic anemia which is associated with aplasia of the bone marrow is characterized by a reduction in the peripheral blood of erythrocytes, white cells and platelets. About 50 percent of cases are the result of exposure to ionizing radiation or to drugs such as chloramphenicol, anticonvulsants, antimalarials and gold compounds, while in the remainder no cause can be found (idiopathic aplastic anemia).

CLINICAL FEATURES. The patient may complain of weakness due to anemia or may present with hemorrhagic manifestations because of the lowered platelet count. In patients with marked leukopenia, the first symptom may be a severe infection. Examination will reveal pallor and purpura. Bone marrow examination shows fatty replacement of myeloid and erythroid elements.

TREATMENT. Blood transfusions are given. If a drug is found to be the cause of the condition, administration of it is stopped. Steroids are of value in the treatment of the hemorrhagic manifestations. Antibiotics are used to control infection.

### Polycythemia Vera

In this condition, there is a neoplastic increase in the red-cell forming tissue in the bone marrow.

CLINICAL FEATURES. It occurs in the older age group and is associated with an enlarged spleen. The color of the skin is bluish-red and the patient may complain of headache, lassitude and breathlessness. Hemorrhage may occur from the alimentary tract, nose or mouth and excessive bleeding may follow tooth extraction. The red cell count varies from 6 to 10 millions per cubic millimeter. The white cell and platelet counts also rise. Some of these patients ultimately die of leukemia. In 10 percent of cases, there is an underlying renal neoplasm, cyst or hydronephrosis.

TREATMENT is with radioactive phosphorus.

## CONDITIONS AFFECTING THE WHITE BLOOD CELLS

The normal white cell count in the adult varies between 4000 and 10,000 per cubic millimeter. In the first two or three years of life lymphocytes

TABLE 7.2. NORMAL ADULT CIRCULATING LEUKOCYTE COUNTS

| Cell Type | Range of Normal Values | |
| --- | --- | --- |
| | Percent | Per cu. mm. |
| Neutrophils | 40–70 | 1600–7000 |
| Lymphocytes | 20–45 | 800–4500 |
| Monocytes | 2–8 | 80–800 |
| Eosinophils | 0–5 | 0–500 |
| Basophils | 0–1 | 0–100 |

make up 60 percent or more of the circulating leukocytes. By the age of four the circulating lymphocyte and granulocyte counts are about equal; granulocytes then become more numerous and the normal adult distribution is reached by the age of 14 or 15.

A circulating white cell count in excess of 10,000 per cubic millimeter is termed leukocytosis and occurs in a number of infections; a count below 4000 per cubic millimeter is known as leukopenia. In leukopenia the neutrophils are more frequently disproportionately low in which case the term neutropenia or granulocytopenia is best applied.

Leukocytosis accompanies:

1. *Acute infections* especially with pyogenic bacteria
2. *Leukemia*
3. *Diseases associated with acute inflammation or necrosis* as in infarction and collagen diseases
4. *Neoplasms*—carcinoma, lymphoma, especially with areas of tissue necrosis and widespread metastases
5. *Acute hemorrhage*

Leukopenia accompanies:

1. *Infections.* These include typhoid, acute viral infections such as measles and infectious hepatitis, malaria and overwhelming infections such as septicemia
2. *Bone marrow damage.* Irradiation, toxic drugs and chemicals such as benzol and nitrogen mustards, and hypersensitivity to aminopyrine, sulfonamides and chloramphenicol may cause aplastic anemia or neutropenia
3. *Nutritional deficiency.* Vitamin $B_{12}$ and folic acid deficiencies
4. *Blood diseases.* There is a stage in acute leukemia, aleukemic leukemia, in which the white cell count is extremely low

## Cyclic Neutropenia

This is a rare disease of unknown etiology which is characterized by reduction in the number of circulating neutrophils at regular intervals of two to four weeks associated with recurrent oral ulceration.

## Agranulocytosis

This condition is a severe form of leukopenia with fulminating clinical manifestations. It may occur following the administration of drugs such as aminopyrine, sulfonamides, gold or chloramphenicol.

CLINICAL FEATURES. The patient develops severe ulceration of the mouth and fauces with little inflammatory reaction around the ulcers. Because of the reduction of the number of neutrophils, the patient has a diminished resistance to infection and may die.

TREATMENT. Repeated blood transfusions with large doses of penicillin daily to control secondary infection.

## Leukemia

Leukemia is the malignant proliferation of the precursors of white cells in the bone marrow resulting in large numbers of white cells in the peripheral blood, many of which are immature. The etiology is unknown. Leukemias will be classified here into the acute and chronic forms. The former is usually fatal within a few weeks or months and the latter may persist for one or more years before the patient succumbs. The diagnosis is made from examination of the peripheral blood and sternal marrow.

### ACUTE LEUKEMIA

The lymphocytic, myelocytic and monocytic forms have been described but it may be impossible cytologically to distinguish between the different forms. For this reason, a diagnosis of acute leukemia may have to be made without labelling the specific type.

CLINICAL FEATURES. The patient feels unwell and is pale and has the associated syptoms of anemia. Purpuric rashes and hemorrhages from the nose, gingivae and gastrointestinal tract occur. The gingivae are swollen, bluish red and tender and often there may be an associated Vincent's infection due to the lowered resistance. In the lymphocytic and monocytic forms, gingival hypertrophy is often found (Figure 7.5). Histologically, the gingival tissues are packed with immature white cells; the specific type

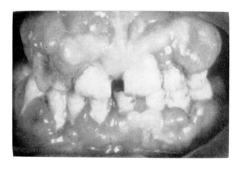

**Figure 7.5.** Monocytic leukemia. The gingivae are pale and hypertrophied and have bled spontaneously on a number of occasions. Male, aged 35 years.

depends on the type of leukemia. The lymph nodes of the neck are enlarged in the presence of oral sepsis and the spleen may be palpable.

TREATMENT. Repeated blood transfusions, antineoplastic drugs and cortisone have been used to produce remissions. Antibiotics are given to control secondary infection.

## CHRONIC MYELOCYTIC LEUKEMIA

The patient feels unwell and shows the symptoms of anemia. Hemorrhages may occur from the gingivae or nose. The spleen is greatly enlarged.

TREATMENT is radiotherapy and chemotherapy using antineoplastic agents.

## CHRONIC LYMPHOCYTIC LEUKEMIA

This is a disease of later life and is more common in males than females. Clinically, the lymph nodes throughout the body are enlarged and the spleen and liver are slightly enlarged. Hemorrhages may occur from the gingivae and gastrointestinal tract. Gingival hypertrophy is less common in chronic leukemia than in the acute varieties. Proliferation of lymphocytes in lacrimal and salivary glands may cause bilateral painless enlargement.

TREATMENT is radiotherapy and also antineoplastic drugs.

# THE PHYSIOLOGY OF BLOOD COAGULATION

## Clotting Factors

The following is a list of the 12 factors which have been recognized as the various substances involved in the coagulation of the blood. There is no factor VI.

Factor I — Fibrinogen
Factor II — Prothrombin
Factor III — Tissue thromboplastin
Factor IV — Calcium
Factor V — Proaccelerin, labile factor
Factor VII — Proconvertin, serum prothrombin conversion accelerator (SPCA), stable factor
Factor VIII — Antihemophilic globulin (AHG)
Factor IX — Plasma thromboplastin component (PTC), Christmas factor
Factor X — Stuart factor, Stuart-Prower factor
Factor XI — Plasma thromboplastin antecedent (PTA)
Factor XII — Hageman factor
Factor XIII — Fibrin stabilizing factor (FSF), fibrinase

## The Three Stages of the Clotting Mechanism

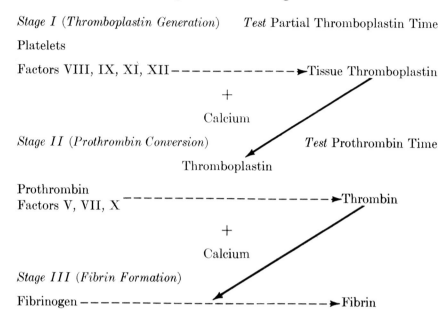

*Stage I (Thromboplastin Generation)*       *Test* Partial Thromboplastin Time

Platelets

Factors VIII, IX, XI, XII – – – – – – – – – – –➤Tissue Thromboplastin

$$+$$

Calcium

*Stage II (Prothrombin Conversion)*          *Test* Prothrombin Time

Thromboplastin

Prothrombin
Factors V, VII, X – – – – – – – – – – – – – – – – – – –➤Thrombin

$$+$$

Calcium

*Stage III (Fibrin Formation)*

Fibrinogen – – – – – – – – – – – – – – – – – – – – –➤Fibrin

# CLINICAL TESTS EMPLOYED IN THE INVESTIGATION OF DISEASES OF THE BLOOD

The whole blood clotting time, one-stage prothrombin time and partial thromboplastin time are tests of plasma clotting activity in common use. The bleeding time, platelet count, tourniquet test and clot retraction test are believed to measure platelet function.

## Tests of Clotting Function

### WHOLE BLOOD CLOTTING TIME

Venous blood is used in preference to "fingerprick" samples which contain admixed tissue elements. A prolonged clotting time indicates that a problem exists which should be further investigated. A normal clotting time does not always ensure that hemostasis is normal.

### ONE-STAGE PROTHROMBIN TIME

This is a test for Stage II defects. A commercial thromboplastin and calcium are mixed with the patient's plasma. The time for the clot to form is recorded and compared with a normal control plasma. The prothrombin time is the procedure of choice in the control of patients receiving hypo-thrombinemic drugs.

## PARTIAL THROMBOPLASTIN TIME (PTT)

This is a one-stage test for Stage I defects. If normal amounts of Factors VIII and IX are present in the plasma, clotting occurs in the normal range which varies with the laboratory. If one of these factors is lacking, the time will be prolonged. It is the usual practice for the laboratory to state its own PTT control in order that one can compare the patient's PTT with that time.

### Tests of Platelet Function

## BLEEDING TIME

This test measures the time necessary for active bleeding to cease from a clean, superficial wound. The Duke method and Ivy method are the tests in general use. Patients with von Willebrand's disease (see p. 101) characteristically have long bleeding times. In hemophilia the bleeding time is normal.

## PLATELET COUNT

The range is from 150,000 to 450,000/cu.mm. The platelet count is decreased in thrombocytopenic purpura.

## TOURNIQUET TEST

This is a nonspecific test for both capillary fragility and platelet function. It measures the ability of the capillary to withstand the stress of increased intraluminal pressure.

A blood pressure cuff is placed on the upper arm and inflated to the mid-point between systolic and diastolic pressure. It is left for five minutes after which the forearm is examined for petechiae. Normal individuals have 0 to 10 petechiae; between 10 and 20 is equivocal; more than 20 indicates abnormal hemostatic function.

## CLOT RETRACTION TEST

Platelet function can be measured conveniently by the clot retraction test. A test tube of blood, without anticoagulant is placed in the incubator at 37° C. The clot should begin to retract in 30 minutes and should be retracted completely in 12 hours.

A failure of the clot to retract indicates either a depressed number of platelets or a failure of the platelets to break up and initiate the clotting process.

### Investigation of Anemia

The red cell count, white cell count, differential white cell count, the hemoglobin and hematocrit levels should be performed routinely.

# THE HEMORRHAGIC DISORDERS

The prevention of spontaneous hemorrhage and undue blood loss from injured vessels is dependent on the integrity of the vessels themselves, on the blood platelets and on the coagulation mechanism. The larger blood vessels react to injury by immediate vasoconstriction and the resultant slowing of the blood flow assists in the agglutination of platelets. The platelets release serotonin (5-hydroxytryptamine) which causes not only a local but also a temporary, general vasoconstriction. In addition, they and the damaged tissues release substances which initiate coagulation.

Disorders of the hemostatic mechanism can be discussed under the headings:

1. Disorders of the vessels themselves
2. Disorders of the platelets
3. Disorders of the coagulation mechanism

## Disorders of the Blood Vessels

The capillary fragility test (tourniquet test) and the bleeding time give some indication of the vascular resistance to injury.

### HEREDITARY HEMORRHAGIC TELANGIECTASIA

This disease, which is rare, is characterized by the development of thin-walled dilatations (telangiectases) of arterioles and capillaries; if injured, they do not contract like normal blood vessels and the result is persistent bleeding. The disease which is inherited as a simple dominant occurs in families and affects the sexes equally.

Telangiectases occur commonly on the face, in the mouth and conjunctivae although any organ may be involved. They appear as blue to bluish-red lesions of variable size. Bleeding can be controlled by pressure.

### PURPURA

Purpura is defined as hemorrhages into the skin and joints and from mucous membranes. It may result from a decrease in the number of platelets, thrombocytopenic purpura. In some conditions, the platelets are normal but hemorrhages result from capillary fragility, vascular purpura. The latter occurs in hereditary hemorrhagic telangiectasia, in senile and anaphylactoid purpura, von Willebrand's disease and scurvy (Figure 7.6).

### Senile Purpura

This condition occurs over the age of 60 years. Purpuric areas are found on the backs of the hands and forearms. It is due to atrophy of the skin with loss of support of the vessels. The condition is not usually associated with excessive bleeding following tooth extraction.

### Anaphylactoid Purpura (Henoch-Schönlein Purpura)

This condition is due to a widespread vasculitis associated with hypersensitivity. It occurs mainly in children and young adults. It may be pre-

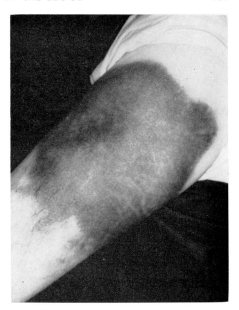

**Figure 7.6.** Thrombocytopenic purpura. There is extensive bruising of the
arm occurring after the patient banged
into a door. Platelet count 10,000 per
cu. mm. Male, aged 40 years.

ceded by a hemolytic streptococcal infection. Purpuric patches occur on
the skin. Hemorrhages may occur into the joints and gastrointestinal
tract.

TREATMENT. Steroid therapy is of value.

### Vascular Hemophilia (von Willebrand's Disease)

This condition is an inherited condition which affects capillaries. It
occurs more frequently in women than in men. Epistaxis and spontaneous
bleeding from the gingivae may occur. Hemorrhage in some cases may
follow cuts or dental extractions. In many cases of von Willebrand's
disease there is an associated deficiency of antihemophilic globulin. The
bleeding time is prolonged and there is often increased capillary fragility.
Bleeding can be controlled by pressure.

### Scurvy (see page 150.)

## Disorders of the Platelets

The platelets may be deficient in quantity (thrombocytopenia) or they
may be defective in function (thrombasthenia). The normal platelet
count is 150,000 to 450,000/cu.mm. and thrombocytopenia is said to occur
when the count is below 100,000/cu.mm. In severe cases of thrombocytopenia, capillary resistance is almost always decreased but this may be due
to damage by the thrombocytopenic agent. Thrombocytopenia may be
induced by sensitivity to drugs such as quinidine and sulfonamides or by
an infection. Often no cause can be detected and this condition is known as

idiopathic thrombocytopenic purpura. The bleeding time is prolonged in thrombocytopenic purpura. Splenectomy usually cures this condition.

### Disorders of the Coagulation Mechanism

The two most common disorders of coagulation are:

1. Hemophilia (antihemophilic globulin deficiency, Factor VIII deficiency)
2. Christmas disease (Christmas factor deficiency, Factor IX deficiency)

The treatment of hemorrhage occurring in a hemophiliac patient demands fresh blood or plasma since Factor VIII is labile on storage. Factor IX deficiency can be treated with ordinary banked plasma. The danger of using large quantities of blood and plasma is that the circulation may be overloaded. For this reason, blood and plasma products are now being employed. Glycine-precipitated antihemophilic globulin (AHG) and cryoprecipitate AHG are now the two products most commonly used in the treatment of hemophilia.

## HEMOPHILIA (FACTOR VIII DEFICIENCY)

This hereditary disease occurs in males but is transmitted by the female. It is due to a deficiency of AHG, Factor VIII, in the plasma leading to deficient formation of thromboplastin.

CLINICAL FEATURES. Hemorrhages occur into the skin and joints following trivial injury and spontaneous bleeding may occur from the nose or gingivae. The hemorrhages into joints may result in crippling osteoarthritis.

## INDICATIONS FOR REPLACEMENT THERAPY OF AHG

Spontaneous bleeding will normally cease when the Factor VIII level is increased to about 15 percent of normal. Control of traumatic bleeding requires a level of 30 to 40 percent of the normal average. For a highly critical hemorrhage such as intracranial hemorrhage or major surgery a level of 50 percent may be necessary. Tooth extraction is an indication for replacement therapy.

## CHRISTMAS DISEASE

This condition which is due to lack of Christmas factor (Factor IX) is inherited in a similar manner to hemophilia. Lack of Christmas factor causes deficient production of thromboplastin.

CLINICAL FEATURES. Christmas disease resembles hemophilia clinically. The first sign of the disease may be excessive bleeding following tonsillectomy or tooth extraction.

EXTRACTION OF TEETH. To prevent hemorrhage following tooth extraction frozen plasma or blood may be used as the Christmas factor does not deteriorate on storage.

## The Effects of Blood Loss

The effects of a hemorrhage are dependent on the amount, location and rate. In a healthy person the loss of 500 ml. of blood produces almost no symptoms but it does lower the hemoglobin eight percent. An anemic patient does not withstand the loss of blood well. Depending on the rate of blood loss hemorrhage may be acute or chronic. Acute blood loss is discussed below. Chronic blood loss leads to hypochromic anemia.

## Acute Hemorrhage

Acute hemorrhage may be severe enough to produce peripheral circulatory failure (shock) and death. In those patients who survive, several compensatory mechanisms occur.

CLINICAL FEATURES. An acute hemorrhage lowers the blood pressure and results in increased cardiac rate and peripheral vasoconstriction. The pulse and respiration are rapid. The skin is pale, cold and moist, and the patient may feel nauseated or faint.

LABORATORY FINDINGS. Immediately following a hemorrhage, hematologic examination will show no decrease in the number of cells because comparable amounts of plasma and cells are lost. A few hours later as dilution of blood occurs with the movement of fluid from the tissues into the capillaries the erythrocyte count, the hemoglobin and hematocrit fall progressively. An increase in reticulocytes occurs and circulating nucleated red cells appear within 24 to 48 hours after an episode of bleeding. Erythrocyte count, hemoglobin and hematocrit will be normal within three to six weeks.

A neutrophil leucocytosis of 10,000 to 20,000/cu. mm. and increased platelet count of 500,000 to 1,000,000/cu.mm. develop within a few hours and persist for several days after the bleeding ceases.

TREATMENT. The hemorrhage is arrested, morphine is given for the treatment of shock and blood transfusion is employed for restoration of the blood volume.

# BLOOD GROUPS
## ABO System

Red cells are grouped into the major ABO categories by testing for the presence of the A and B antigens using the appropriate antisera. Group A individuals have anti-B antibody in their serum; Group B individuals have anti-A. Persons whose red cells are group O have both anti-A and anti-B, those with group AB cells have neither antibody in the serum.

SUBGROUPS OF A. Twenty percent of group A individuals are group $A_2$ and these persons can only receive $A_2$ blood. They cannot receive the more frequent $A_1$ antigen since they have an anti-$A_1$ antibody and hemolysis occurs.

## Rh System

Eighty-five percent of the white population has a red cell antigen which agglutinates a rabbit antiserum prepared against the cells of rhesus monkeys. Patients who possess this red cell antigen are rhesus-positive. The remaining 15 percent of the population lacks this rhesus factor and is termed rhesus-negative.

There are five major antigens in the Rh system and $Rh_o$, also named D, is the most important. Members of the 15 percent of the population who lack this antigen can if transfused with cells containing the antigen be easily stimulated to form an anti-$Rh_o$ (D) antibody. Antibodies, once formed, persist for many years so that transfusion at a later date may result in a transfusion reaction. Rh-negative women should not receive Rh-positive blood because of the danger of hemolytic disease of the newborn.

## HEMOLYTIC DISEASE OF THE NEWBORN

An Rh-negative woman who bears an Rh-positive fetus will develop anti-Rh antibodies. In subsequent pregnancies various degrees of hemolysis may occur in the fetal blood. The most severely affected infants die in utero (hydrops fetalis). The symptoms vary in milder cases but usually the spleen and liver are enlarged and jaundice appears soon after birth. Blood destruction continuing after birth causes progressive anemia and hyperbilirubinemia. If circulating bilirubin rises to $>20$ mg./100 ml. it may produce kernicterus (bile staining of the basal ganglia) which is characterized by muscular twitching or convulsions. If untreated these children show mental retardation and spasticity.

### Other Blood Groups

There are other blood groups which can cause clinical problems. The most important are the Kell (K), Duffy (Fy) and Lewis. Antibodies for these agglutinins can be demonstrated by the Coombs test.

### TRANSFUSION THERAPY

Blood transfusion is not without danger. Transfusion reaction, the infusion of incompatible blood, is the most serious; intravascular hemolysis occurs and may be fatal. Other risks are febrile or allergic reactions; transmission of infectious diseases such as hepatitis, syphilis and malaria or stimulation of antibody production which might complicate later transfusions or childbearing.

### GENERAL REFERENCES

Goodale, R. H. and Widmann, F. K.: *Clinical Interpretation of Laboratory Tests*, 6th ed., Philadelphia, Davis, 1969.
Linman, J. W.: *Principles of Hematology*, New York, Macmillan, 1966.

### SUGGESTED READING

Monti, A.: "Diseases of the blood and blood-forming organs" in *Internal Medicine Based on Mechanisms of Disease* (Eds. P. J. Talso and A. P. Remenchik), St. Louis, Mosby, 1968, pp. 644–694.
*Proceedings Dental Hemophilia Institute*, The National Hemophilia Foundation, January, 1968.

## CHAPTER 8

# DISEASES OF THE LYMPH NODES

Enlargement of the lymph nodes (lymphadenopathy) may conveniently be divided into localized and generalized enlargements and the causes of these are as follows:

**Localized Enlargement**

1. Acute lymphadenitis
2. Tuberculous lymphadenitis
3. Non-specific chronic lymphadenitis
4. Secondary carcinoma

It should be noted that a lymph node may enlarge during an acute infection and may remain enlarged after the infection has subsided; this condition is termed non-specific chronic lymphadenitis. The causes of localized enlargement are covered in textbooks of surgery.

**Generalized Enlargement**

1. Rubella (p. 4)
2. Infectious mononucleosis (p. 9)
3. Secondary syphilis (p. 11)
4. Still's disease (p. 156)
5. Chronic lymphocytic leukemia (p. 97)
6. Reticulum cell sarcoma
7. Lymphosarcoma
8. Hodgkin's disease
9. Follicular lymphoma

The last four are tumors of lymphatic tissue or lymphomas and are dealt with below.

## TUMORS OF LYMPHATIC TISSUE (LYMPHOMAS)

The lymphomas are the most common form of malignant tumor after the carcinomas. With the possible exception of Burkitt's lymphoma their etiology is unknown. They arise from the cellular elements of the lymph nodes and bone marrow and, unlike other types of sarcoma, they spread rapidly to other lymph nodes. Initially the nodes are discrete and freely movable but may become matted and fixed as surrounding structures are invaded. Lymphomatous nodes are firm and rubbery in consistency. The spleen, liver and bone marrow are extensively infiltrated and lymphomatous deposits are also present in the lungs and other organs.

TREATMENT. The lymphomas are extremely radiosensitive; dramatic remissions follow radiotherapy. Sometimes a localized lesion may be cured but, unfortunately, recurrence and spread to other lymph nodes are the rule.

In general, surgery is useful in the treatment of lymphomas when the condition is localized; x-ray therapy is effective in the treatment of local manifestations and when the disease is generalized, and chemotherapy is valuable when the disorder is widespread. The most effective chemotherapeutic agents are nitrogen mustard, chlorambucil and cyclophosphamide.

### Reticulum Cell Sarcoma (Reticulosarcoma)

This tumor arises from the primitive reticulum cells scattered throughout the lymph nodes. These cells lay down reticulin fibers and may assume a fibroblastic activity, with resulting deposition of collagen. In reticulum cell sarcoma, the normal architecture of the node is obliterated by large neoplastic reticulum cells.

Reticulosarcoma usually starts in a group of lymph nodes or, more rarely, in a tonsil and soon involves the spleen and liver which become clinically palpable.

### Lymphosarcoma

Lymphosarcoma is clinically indistinguishable from reticulum cell sarcoma. Histologic examination shows infiltration of the lymph nodes with neoplastic lymphocytes. A special variety is *Burkitt's lymphoma*, a lymphosarcoma occurring in certain parts of Africa. It occurs almost exclusively in children between the ages of two and fourteen years and affects the jaws (especially the maxilla), ovaries, retroperitoneal lymph nodes and kidneys. The herpes-like virus (HLV) is suspected of playing a part in the pathogenesis of Burkitt's lymphoma and, in addition, in carcinoma of the posterior nasal space and infectious mononucleosis.

## Hodgkin's Disease

The most common lymphoma is found in Hodgkin's disease which attacks young and middle-aged adults predominantly. Histologic examination shows replacement of the affected lymph nodes by a number of different types of cells, the most important of which are neoplastic reticulum cells. These vary in size and shape and include in their number giant cells with double, mirror-image nuclei (Sternberg-Reed giant cells). The other cells present include lymphocytes, plasma cells, neutrophils and often many eosinophils.

Hodgkin's disease usually presents with a localized enlargement of lymph nodes and the patient is usually free of symptoms at this stage. The cervical lymph nodes are most commonly involved especially those in the posterior triangle (Figure 8.1). If the patient is left untreated, further enlargement of the original group of glands together with the appearance of enlarged nodes elsewhere is the rule. General symptoms may now appear and these include fever, lassitude, anorexia, loss of weight, pruritus (itching of the skin), pain in the chest and abdomen, dyspnea and cough. The patient at this stage may appear wasted with pigmentation of the skin and anemia, painless enlargement of lymph nodes, and an enlarged spleen and liver. If the disease is unchecked, bleeding, jaundice, neurologic complications and severe infection by opportunist microorganisms are frequent causes of death.

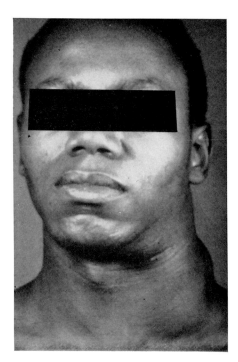

**Figure 8.1.** Hodgkin's disease. There is marked enlargement of the cervical lymph nodes. Diagnosis confirmed by histologic examination of a node. Male, aged 27 years.

A much less malignant variety called *paragranuloma* also occurs. It remains localized for a long time and can be cured by radiotherapy. The node is replaced by masses of mature lymphocytes among which are the Sternberg-Reed giant cells. If all age groups are taken together, 40 percent of patients with Hodgkin's disease will be alive after 15 years.

### Follicular Lymphoma

Follicular lymphoma is the least common of the four lymphomas and, like paragranuloma, runs a slow course. Histologic examination shows replacement of the node by a dense mass of giant lymphocytic follicles distributed uniformly throughout its substance. The condition eventually terminates in lymphosarcoma or reticulum cell sarcoma.

## DENTAL IMPLICATIONS OF LYMPH NODE ENLARGEMENT

Acute infections of the pulp and periodontium will usually result in tender enlargement of the submandibular lymph nodes. Patients with acute herpetic stomatitis and acute necrotizing gingivitis will frequently complain of enlarged and tender cervical lymph nodes. The tenderness will subside with improvement of the infection. However, they may remain palpable for some months after the acute symptoms have disappeared. Penicillin is the antibiotic of choice for most dental infections with the exception of acute herpetic stomatitis (see p. 5). When the patient is sensitive to penicillin, erythromycin is prescribed.

Infections of the tonsil will produce enlargement of the lymph node situated at the angle of the mandible, the jugulodigastric or tonsillar lymph

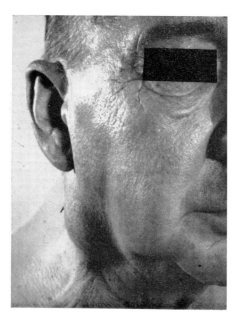

**Figure 8.2.** Metastatic carcinoma. The cervical lymph nodes are involved by metastases from a squamous cell carcinoma of the tonsil. The diagnosis was confirmed histologically. Male, aged 57 years.

node. Patients with acute tonsillitis may complain of pain on certain movements of the head which trap the enlarged node beneath the angle of the mandible.

In any patient presenting with acute enlargement of the cervical lymph nodes a focus of infection should be sought on the scalp, on the face, in the external auditory meatus, in the vestibule of the nose and in the oral cavity. On occasion an acutely inflamed lymph node may suppurate and require incision and drainage.

Secondary carcinoma is the commonest cause of a chronic lymph node swelling in the neck over the age of 50. The swelling is firm on palpation and, except in early cases, fixed (Figure 8.2).

## SUGGESTED READING

Annotation. Outlook in Hodgkin's Disease. Brit. Med. J., *2*, 328, 1967.
Linman, J. W.: *Principles of Hematology*, New York, Macmillan, 1966, pp. 380–410.
Woodruff, M. F. A.: *Surgery for Dental Students*, 2nd ed., Oxford, Blackwell Scientific Publications, 1966, pp. 229–237.

## CHAPTER 9

# DISEASES OF THE SALIVARY GLANDS

It is proposed to discuss in this chapter some of the nonsurgical conditions of the three paired major salivary glands: the parotids, submandibular and sublingual glands. A convenient classification of diseases of the salivary glands is as follows:

**Inflammatory Conditions**

ACUTE
1. Bacterial: parotid abscess
2. Viral: mumps (p. 8)

CHRONIC
1. Sialectasis
2. Sialolithiasis
3. Tuberculosis
4. Actinomycosis
5. Sarcoidosis (p. 37)

**Autoimmune Disease**

1. Sjögren's syndrome
2. Benign lymphoepithelial lesion (Mikulicz's disease)

**Allergy and Drug Reactions**

**Metabolic Conditions**

1. Cirrhosis of the liver
2. Malnutrition

**Disorders of Salivation**

1. Xerostomia
2. Sialorrhea
3. Drooling

**Neoplasms**

## AUTOIMMUNE DISEASE

### Sjögren's Syndrome

Sjögren's syndrome is currently regarded as an autoimmune disease. Histologically the parotid and lacrimal glands show round cell infiltration and atrophy of the glandular tissue. Because the histologic picture is similar to benign lymphoepithelial lesion (Mikulicz's disease) it is now believed that the two conditions are related.

CLINICAL FEATURES. Sjögren's syndrome occurs predominantly in middle-aged females. The patient complains of a dry mouth (xerostomia), inability to produce tears (keratoconjunctivitis sicca) and rheumatoid arthritis or, rarely, other connective tissue diseases such as systemic lupus erythematosus, polyarteritis nodosa, progressive systemic sclerosis and polymyositis. The term "sicca syndrome" is used to describe the combina-

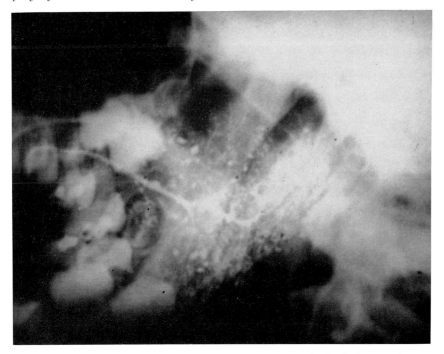

**Figure 9.1.** Sjögren's disease. A sialogram of the parotid gland shows sialectasis which represents radiopaque material situated within dilatations of the terminal ducts. Female, aged 54 years.

tion of oral and ocular manifestations and these two components of the triad are generally considered sufficient for the diagnosis.

The parotid glands in the early stages of the disease are slightly enlarged but later in the disease no swelling is observed. Parotid sialography reveals dilatation of the terminal ducts (sialectasis) of variable degree (Figure 9.1).

Atrophy of the oral mucosa may be observed. Because of the reduced salivary flow there may be an increased caries incidence.

LABORATORY DIAGNOSIS. Leukopenia and eosinophilia are common findings. Tests for rheumatoid factor using human gamma globulin as antigen are positive in nearly 100 percent of patients. LE cells, antinuclear factor, complement fixing and precipitating antibodies may also be found in some patients. Biopsy of labial mucous glands is used to confirm the diagnosis of Sjögren's syndrome.

TREATMENT. This is symptomatic. To relieve the dry mouth, one percent methyl cellulose mouthwash may be used as frequently as required. Methyl cellulose 0.5 percent eyedrops are instilled two or three times daily as artificial tears.

### Benign Lymphoepithelial Lesion (Mikulicz's Disease)

In 1888 Mikulicz reported a male patient with massive enlargement of the lacrimal, parotid and submandibular glands but without xerostomia or xerophthalmia. Biopsy of the glands showed massive round cell infiltration and atrophy of the acinar parenchyma. As stated above, this condition is now thought to be related to Sjögren's syndrome.

## ALLERGY AND DRUG REACTIONS

Allergic swelling of the parotids and occasionally of the submandibular glands has been reported in middle-aged women with a history of asthma or hayfever. Antihistamines are of little value in treatment.

Swelling of the parotids has been described following administration of butazolidin in sensitive patients.

## METABOLIC CONDITIONS

Enlargement of the parotids has been reported in cirrhosis of the liver and malnutrition.

It should be remembered that whenever there is stasis within the parotid gland there is the possibility of an ascending infection via the parotid duct.

## DISORDERS OF SALIVATION

Patients may occasionally complain of dry mouth (xerostomia) or of excessive salivation (sialorrhea). These two symptoms will now be discussed.

### Xerostomia

The following conditions can result in xerostomia:

## CONGENITAL APLASIA OF ONE OR MORE SALIVARY GLANDS

This is an extremely rare cause of dry mouth.

## ADMINISTRATION OF DRUGS

Patients who are taking atropine, chlorpromazine and some of the appetite suppressants may complain of dry mouth. It is essential to question any patient who complains of xerostomia if he is receiving any medication, and if so, the name of the drug so that its pharmacologic activity can be checked.

## SYSTEMIC DISEASES

In fever, uncontrolled diabetes and Sjögren's syndrome, xerostomia is frequently present.

## PHYSIOLOGIC CONDITIONS

In menopause and old age the patient may complain of a dry mouth.

## PSYCHIC FACTORS

In fear and anxiety a common symptom is xerostomia.

## INJURIES TO THE SALIVARY GLANDS

Patients who have had irradiation of the salivary glands complain of a dry mouth. In some patients extensive caries occurs because of the reduced salivary flow.

### Sialorrhea

Excessive salivation can be discussed under the following headings:

## CHILDHOOD

Salivary flow is characteristically greater in infancy and early childhood. In "teething" sialorrhea may be observed.

## ADMINISTRATION OF DRUGS

Pilocarpine, iodides, ammonium and mercurial salts cause excessive salivation.

## STOMATITIS

In all types of stomatitis whether due to infection or an unknown etiology such as erythema multiforme, pemphigus and pemphigoid there is increased salivation.

## INSERTION OF PROSTHETIC APPLIANCES

Any prosthetic appliance when first inserted into the mouth acts as a foreign body and stimulates salivation. When the patient is accustomed to the appliance, increased salivation is no longer a problem.

## Drooling

It is important to distinguish sialorrhea from drooling. The latter results from failure to swallow salivary secretions or from inability to retain the accumulated secretions within the mouth because of a seventh-nerve palsy or facial disfigurement. It is the difference between salivary production and the ability to swallow saliva that results in drooling rather than the quantity of saliva produced.

Difficulty in swallowing saliva may occur as a result of defects of deglutition at the oral, pharyngeal and esophageal levels. Some common disorders associated with drooling, classified according to the presumable level of malfunction, are: oral (cerebral palsy, Parkinsonism, seventh-nerve palsy, motor-neuron disease and radical neck surgery); pharyngeal (motor-neuron disease and myasthenia gravis); and esophageal (carcinoma or stricture).

## NEOPLASMS

The major salivary glands are involved by both benign and malignant neoplasms and these are adequately covered in textbooks of oral pathology and general surgery.

## SUGGESTED READING

SJÖGREN'S SYNDROME
Bloch, K. J., Buchanan, W. W., Wohl, M. J., and Bunim, J. J.: Sjögren's syndrome. A clinical, pathological, and serological study of sixty-two cases. Medicine, *44*, 187, 1965.

ALLERGY AND THE PAROTID
Cohen, L.: Recurrent swelling of the parotid gland. Report of a case due to allergy. Brit. Dent. J., *118*, 487, 1964.

DRUG REACTIONS AND THE PAROTID
Cohen, L. and Banks, P. L.: Salivary gland enlargement and phenylbutazone (butazolidin). Brit. Med. J., *1*, 1420, 1966.

PAROTID ENLARGEMENT
Maynard, J.: Parotid enlargement. Hosp. Med., *1*, 620, 1967. (Contains a list of the most important references.)

SIALORRHEA
Smith, R. A. and Goode, R. L.: Sialorrhea. New Eng. J. Med., *283*, 917, 1970.

## Chapter 10

# DISORDERS OF NUTRITION

The term nutrition means the utilization of food derivatives in the growth, maintenance and repair of body tissues and in providing for energy requirements. Diet is the total of all ingested food, both solids and liquids. A satisfactory diet should include carbohydrate, fat, protein, vitamins, water and inorganic elements.

## CARBOHYDRATES

The term "carbohydrate" embraces a wide range of different substances. In nutrition, however, the carbohydrates are considered to be those substances which appear in appreciable quantities in food as simple sugars or are converted to such sugars in the digestive processes. They are classified as monosaccharides, disaccharides and polysaccharides.

### Carbohydrates In the Diet

It has been shown that when the amount of food is adequate, absence of dietary carbohydrate causes fatigue, ketosis and loss of weight. These effects are associated with loss of body water and salt.

### Obesity and Overweight

Obesity is a condition in which there is a disproportionate amount of fat in the body. Diabetic mothers give birth to obese babies and this suggests that disordered carbohydrate metabolism may be an etiologic factor. In addition it is known that high levels of glucose in the blood suppress utilization of fats and lead to their retention.

The overweight person not only has an excessive accumulation of body fat but of other body components as well because of an imbalance between the amount of food ingested and the energy expended. Weight reduction is best achieved by an overall reduction of the diet rather than by a reduction in the amount of carbohydrates ingested.

## Carbohydrate and Dental Disease

An association between carbohydrate in the diet and dental caries has been established. However, no relationship has been established in man between periodontal disease and the nutritional value of the diet.

## FAT

Fat has a calorie content more than twice that in carbohydrate or protein of equivalent weight. Dietary fat delays gastric emptying and thus delays the onset of the sensation of hunger. The bulk of the fat eaten is in the form of triglyceride. Other important lipids are the fat-soluble vitamins and cholesterol of which the latter has been implicated in the etiology of atherosclerosis.

It has been shown in man that polyunsaturated fats lower a raised serum cholesterol level, whereas saturated fats raise the level. Sufficient evidence is available to show that myocardial infarction in young and middle-aged men can be postponed or prevented by reduction of the intake of animal fats and replacement by vegetable and fish fats and oils.

## PROTEIN

The protein requirement for a normal adult is 1 Gm. per day for each kilogram of body weight. A child, however, needs more protein in proportion to body weight to allow for growth which is most rapid during the first year of life. Increased protein is also required in pregnancy and lactation.

Adults who are fed on a protein-deficient diet become wasted, hypoproteinemic and eventually edematous, the so-called famine edema. In tropical countries where meat and milk are scarce and expensive, protein deficiency occurs among recently weaned children. This condition is known as kwashiorkor.

## Kwashiorkor

Edema, depigmentation and desquamation of skin, apathy and gross fatty enlargement of the liver occur. The treatment is to give a diet consisting mainly of milk.

## VITAMINS

The vitamins which are present in the diet in minute amounts aid in maintaining the normal activities of the tissues. They are divided into the fat-soluble and water-soluble vitamins. The fat-soluble vitamins are

A, D, E and K. The water-soluble vitamins include vitamin C, thiamine, niacin, riboflavin, pyridoxine, pantothenic acid, biotin, folic acid and cyanocobalamin.

## Fat-Soluble Vitamins

### VITAMIN A

Vitamin A is a fat-soluble vitamin which is found chiefly in fish-liver oils, milk and egg yolk; it is stored principally in the liver. This vitamin is necessary for the maintenance of epithelial tissues in a normal condition. The retinal rods and cones are light receptors. The outer segment of both kinds of receptor contain light-sensitive pigments which require vitamin A for their formation and proper functioning. The daily requirement of vitamin A is 1500 I.U. (1.5 mg.) per day.

### Vitamin A Deficiency

One of the first signs is reduced visual acuity in subdued light or night blindness. Extreme deficiency in children results in xerophthalmia (dryness and opacity of the bulbar conjunctiva); Bitot's spots which have a foamy appearance are seen on the lateral margin of the cornea and corneal ulceration may occur. The fundamental change from deficiency of this vitamin is metaplasia of normal nonkeratinized epithelium into a keratinizing type.

TREATMENT. For avitaminosis A, 500,000 I.U. of vitamin A daily for three or more days is recommended.

### Hypervitaminosis A

Intake of vitamin A in excess of 50,000 I.U. daily results in acute toxicity. In children the symptoms are drowsiness, vomiting, bulging of the fontanelles and failure to thrive. Radiographically, new bone formation is present. In adults, headache, blurred vision, nausea, vomiting and bone pains occur. The skin becomes coarse and there is loss of hair.

### VITAMIN D (p. 148)

### VITAMIN E

Vitamin E is present in vegetable oils, wheat germ, corn oil and whole germ. There are three naturally occurring compounds with vitamin E activity, alpha, beta and gamma tocopherol.

### Vitamin E Deficiency

Vitamin E is now known to be essential for humans. Recently a vitamin E responsive megaloblastic anemia in malnourished children has been described (Majaj et al., 1963).

### VITAMIN K

Vitamin K is essential for the formation of prothrombin in the liver. Vitamins $K_1$ and $K_2$ occur naturally and are fat-soluble. Several synthetic naphthoquinone derivatives which have vitamin K activity have been synthesized, including menadione (fat-soluble) and menadione sodium bisulfite (water-soluble). Vitamin K is derived from the diet and synthesis by intestinal bacteria, the latter being the most important source.

### Vitamin K Deficiency

A deficiency of vitamin K causes hypoprothrombinemia which is manifested by defective coagulation of the blood and hemorrhages. For absorption of vitamin K, bile salts are required and for this reason vitamin K deficiency is usually secondary to external biliary fistulas or to obstructive jaundice. In addition, inadequate absorption may occur in other gastrointestinal conditions, including ulcerative colitis and the steatorrheas. In severe liver disease hypoprothrombinemia occurs which does not respond to vitamin K therapy.

### Anticoagulant Drugs

Prothrombin formation in the liver is depressed by bishydroxycoumarin and the other hypoprothrombinemic agents resulting in a prolonged prothrombin time. Heparin acts antagonistically to thrombin, prothrombin and thromboplastin and also decreases the adhesiveness and agglutinability of the platelets.

CLINICAL FEATURES. In vitamin K deficiency hemorrhages may occur from the gingivae, nose or gastrointestinal tract.

LABORATORY FINDINGS. For vitamin K deficiency the prothrombin time of Quick is increased (normal: 10 to 15 seconds). The prothrombin level may also be expressed quantitatively in terms of a percentage of normal (normal: 100 percent). As a rule, bleeding time and coagulation time are little altered until the prothrombin level has fallen to < 20 percent.

TREATMENT. Vitamin $K_1$ (phytonadione) is the drug of choice in reversing the anticoagulant effect of coumarin and indandione derivatives. It is given orally or intramuscularly in doses of 5 to 20 mg. When given intravenously vitamin $K_1$ reverses the effects of anticoagulants within four hours.

## Water-Soluble Vitamins

### VITAMIN C (p. 150)

### THIAMINE (VITAMIN B₁)

Vitamin $B_1$ is found in lean pork, whole grain, enriched bread and cereals, legumes, milk and nuts. It is essential for the proper metabolism of carbohydrates, for the normal functioning of nervous tissue and as part of a series of coenzymes necessary for decarboxylation reactions. Requirement of thiamine is increased in hypothyroidism, pregnancy and febrile conditions.

### Thiamine Deficiency

A deficiency of thiamine results in beriberi.

CLINICAL FEATURES. The symptoms of anorexia, fatigue, poor memory and inability to concentrate precede the neurologic changes. The latter consist of both motor and sensory loss in the feet and legs and later in the arms. In some patients with beriberi edema and cardiac failure occur.

TREATMENT. In mild cases thiamine hydrochloride is given in doses of 10 to 20 mg. by mouth or by injection. In more severe cases up to 200 mg. may be given daily by injection in divided doses.

## NIACIN (NICOTINIC ACID)

Niacin is found in whole grains and enriched bread and cereals, liver, poultry and fish. It is a component of two coenzymes important in glycolysis and tissue respiration. Protein which contains tryptophan protects against a low niacin intake, as tryptophan is a precursor of niacin. The recommended allowances, expressed in niacin equivalents (60 mg. of tryptophan is assumed to be equivalent to 1 mg. niacin) are 6.6 mg./1000 calories.

### Niacin Deficiency

Deficiency of niacin results in pellagra. Primary deficiencies usually are associated with a high-maize diet. Secondary deficiencies frequently occur when there is malabsorption of water-soluble vitamins as in chronic diarrhea.

CLINICAL FEATURES. The classic symptoms of advanced pellagra are scarlet stomatitis and glossitis, diarrhea, dermatitis and mental disturbances such as delirium and psychosis. The skin lesions usually occur on exposed parts and consist of erythema followed by vesiculation and crusting.

TREATMENT. Niacin in daily doses of 300 to 500 mg. are given orally in divided doses.

## RIBOFLAVIN

Good sources of riboflavin are liver, milk, eggs, lean meat, whole grain and enriched cereals. Riboflavin is essential for proper growth and tissue function. The daily riboflavin allowance is computed at the rate of 0.6 mg. per 1000 calories.

### Riboflavin Deficiency

A deficiency of riboflavin in the diet causes macerated lesions at the corners of the mouth (angular cheilosis). Later these lesions may become infected with bacteria or *Candida* and the lesions are then referred to as an angular cheilitis. In addition riboflavin deficiency results in changes in the color and coating of the tongue, redness of the conjunctiva, burning and excessive dryness of the eyes.

9

TREATMENT. Ten to 30 mg. per day are given in divided doses. It should be noted that angular cheilitis rarely responds to riboflavin alone. The application of antibiotic or antifungal ointments is frequently required.

## PYRIDOXINE

Cereals, liver and other meats are good sources of pyridoxine and the related compounds pyridoxal and pyridoxamine. Pyridoxal phosphate functions as the coenzyme for transamination reactions in fatty acid metabolism. The normal adult requirement is 1.5 to 2 mg. per day.

### Pyridoxine Deficiency

This may be induced by consuming a diet deficient in pyridoxine or by administration of a pyridoxine antagonist, deoxypyridoxine. Pyridoxine deprivation in infants results in epileptiform convulsions, impaired growth and a microcytic hypochromic anemia. In adults, cheilosis, conjunctivitis, glossitis and anemia have been described. The peripheral neuropathy sometimes observed during isoniazid therapy of tuberculosis may be prevented or relieved by administration of pyridoxine. Severe alcoholism may also induce pyridoxine deficiency and result in convulsions.

TREATMENT. Five to 10 mg. of pyridoxine are given intramuscularly followed by 1 mg. b.i.d. orally for seven to ten days. During isoniazid therapy 25 to 50 mg. should be given orally.

## PANTOTHENIC ACID

The richest source of pantothenic acid is liver and 10 to 20 mg. per day are recommended. Pantothenic acid is part of coenzyme A which is involved in many acetylation reactions. No characteristic deficiency has been described in man.

## BIOTIN

Biotin is found in egg yolk, liver, most vegetables and fruit. It is believed to function as a coenzyme in metabolism. In man no characteristic symptoms of biotin deficiency have been described.

## FOLIC ACID

Folic acid is found in plentiful supplies in green leafy vegetables, yeast, liver and mushrooms. Vitamin C is essential for the reduction of folic acid to its metabolically active form, tetrahydrofolic acid.

### Folic Acid Deficiency

Alcohol interferes with the intermediary metabolism of folic acid and chronic alcoholics are prone to develop macrocytic anemia from folic acid deficiency. Folic acid deficiency occurs in intestinal malabsorption such as tropical sprue.

CLINICAL FEATURES. The tongue is red, swollen and depapillated. The patient with tropical sprue complains of lassitude, diarrhea and weight loss.

LABORATORY DIAGNOSIS. The peripheral blood shows a macrocytic anemia and the bone marrow shows megaloblastic erythropoiesis instead of the normal precursors of the red cells. The red cells in the peripheral blood show variations in size and shape. In addition leukopenia and reduction of platelets are found. Serum folic acid levels of $< 5$ μg./ml. are diagnostic of deficiency.

TREATMENT. Five mg. of folic acid by mouth daily should produce full therapeutic effects, even in patients with intestinal malabsorption. Although folic acid will produce a hematologic response in pernicious anemia it will not prevent the neurologic manifestations of pernicious anemia and in some cases may accelerate their appearance.

## CYANOCOBALAMIN (VITAMIN B₁₂)

Cyanocobalamin is found in liver and is also produced by the growth of certain microorganisms. For absorption of cyanocobalamin the intrinsic factor of the stomach is necessary and the gastric mucosa fails to secrete this in pernicious anemia (p. 93).

## WATER

Water represents 45 to 75 percent of the total body weight. This percentage varies with the amount of fat: the leaner the individual, the greater the proportion of water to total body weight. Until the age of 12 months, the infant has the highest proportion of body water.

### Loss of Water

Water leaves the body through the kidneys, lungs, skin and gastrointestinal tract. In the normal adult, the gastrointestinal losses are very small. About 1500 ml. of water are lost each day through the kidneys and about 1000 ml. through the skin and lungs. The loss of water via the lungs and skin will increase when there is:

1. Fever
2. An increase in the respiratory rate
3. Hot and dry environment
4. Injury to the skin as in burns.

When there is an increase in dissolved substances in the urine as in diabetes, the kidney has to excrete large quantities of urine in order to carry the increased urinary glucose. In addition, the antidiuretic hormone (ADH) controls the reabsorption of water in the distal convoluted tubules. Increased levels of ADH lead to increased reabsorption of water, which in turn leads to a more concentrated urine.

### Measurement of Water Balance

The simplest and most accurate way to monitor water balance is to determine body weight daily. A weight change of one kilogram (2.2 pounds) equals a fluid loss or gain of one liter.

## The Water Content of the Body

The three body fluid compartments are: intravascular (plasma within the blood vessels), interstitial (fluid within the spaces between cells in the tissues) and intracellular (fluid within the cells). The intravascular and interstitial compartments are usually grouped together as extracellular fluid. The main difference between the plasma and the interstitial fluid is the much higher concentration of protein in plasma. In all other respects the fluids are very similar. The intracellular fluid is characterized by increased potassium, phosphate and protein.

## GASTROINTESTINAL SECRETIONS

About eight liters of saliva, gastric juices and intestinal secretions pass into the gastrointestinal tract each day.

In the healthy person the bulk of these secretions are reabsorbed and are not lost from the body. However, in diarrhea, vomiting, gastrointestinal suction, drainage of fistulas and some malabsorption syndromes large quantities of fluid and electrolytes may be lost. These losses must be made good either by ingestion or intravenous replacement.

## INORGANIC ELEMENTS

### Sodium

Sodium is the principal cation of the extracellular fluids. An increase in the concentration of sodium stimulates the secretion of ADH by the pituitary and results in the retention of water. The average daily intake of NaCl by the adult is 6 to 15 Gm.

## SODIUM EXCRETION

In temperate climates and under normal conditions, sodium loss from the skin is negligible. With increased environmental temperature, fever or muscular exercise the loss of sodium may become quite marked. Under normal conditions the kidney is the chief regulator of sodium in the body. Aldosterone which is secreted by the adrenal cortex inhibits renal sodium excretion. In addition, ADH promotes the reabsorption of water in the distal convoluted tubules and thus has an effect on the concentration of extracellular sodium.

CLINICAL FEATURES. Gastric mucus has a high sodium content and in protracted vomiting large amounts of sodium may be lost. Moreover, chloride is lost in the acid gastric juice. Loss of water and sodium from the plasma is followed by transfer of sodium and water from the interstitial fluid in replacement. Should the loss continue, the water will be removed from the cells. When the plasma volume can no longer be sustained, the function of the circulation will fail. The purpose of intravenous therapy is to restore the normal sodium level.

## Potassium

Potassium is the principal cation of the intracellular fluids.

## POTASSIUM EXCRETION

Potassium is not conserved as well or as promptly by the kidney as sodium. If a patient fails to receive potassium but continues to receive sodium, significant potassium depletion may occur in a normal adult in one week. Both potassium and hydrogen ions compete for exchange with sodium ions in the renal tubules, and adrenal steroids increase urinary potassium loss when sodium is provided.

## INTERNAL CIRCULATION OF POTASSIUM

Potassium is continually moving into and out of cells. The potassium gradient between the intra- and extracellular components is influenced by adrenal steroids, testosterone, pH changes, glycogen formation and hyponatremia (low sodium level).

CLINICAL FEATURES. Increased potassium loss is found in some diseases of the kidney, in metabolic alkalosis (persistent vomiting with substantial loss of hydrochloric acid or from excessive intake of bicarbonates), diabetic acidosis and infantile diarrhea. The minimum daily requirement of potassium is about 40 mEq. However the hospitalized patient receiving intravenous fluids needs 60 to 120 mEq. of potassium daily.

## Calcium

Calcium makes up about 1.5 to 2 percent of the body weight of the human adult, more than 99 percent of it in bones and teeth. Calcium ions also play a role in blood coagulation, neuromuscular irritability, muscle contractility and myocardial function.

The bones act as a reservoir for calcium. When patients are confined to bed, decalcification of the bones occurs and intravenous calcium will not prevent this condition. The blood calcium level is controlled by parathormone (p. 126).

## Magnesium

Magnesium is essential in many enzymatic systems involving carbohydrate, lipid and protein metabolism. It is predominantly an intracellular ion. Most of the ingested magnesium is excreted in the feces.

CLINICAL FEATURES. Magnesium deficiency occurs in severe malabsorption, prolonged nasogastric suction, primary aldosteronism, acute pancreatitis, diabetic acidosis during treatment and chronic alcoholism. The symptoms of magnesium deficiency are muscle tremors, convulsions or delirium.

Magnesium sulfate produces depression of the C.N.S. when given intravenously. Magnesium as well as potassium levels rise in uremia.

## Iron

The normal daily requirement of iron is 10 mg. in males and 15 mg. in females. Good sources of iron are eggs, meat and spinach. Ingested iron is reduced to the ferrous form in the stomach and intestine. It is believed that iron is absorbed as an iron-amino acid complex. The absorbed iron combines with transferrin and is transported to the bone marrow for hemoglobin synthesis or to the body stores. The breakdown of hemoglobin releases iron which is used again and again. Iron is lost from the body during menstruation, pregnancy and lactation.

## IRON DEFICIENCY ANEMIA (p. 92)

## HEMOCHROMATOSIS

Hemochromatosis is characterized by the elevation of plasma iron and increased deposition of iron in the tissues in the form of ferritin and hemosiderin. There are two views of the pathogenesis of hemochromatosis: the classic view is that it is the result of an inborn error of iron metabolism resulting in increased absorption of iron; the other view is that hemochromatosis is a variant of portal cirrhosis.

CLINICAL FEATURES. The skin is pigmented and diabetes, cirrhosis of the liver, testicular atrophy and cardiac disease leading to cardiac failure may occur.

TREATMENT. The patient is bled at weekly intervals to reduce the iron stores. Chelating agents may be given to remove iron.

## Iodine

Iodine is essential for the formation of thyroxine and triiodothyronine (p. 128). Seafood such as fish and oysters are rich in iodine. Iodized table salt is another good source of the element. The minimum daily requirement is 0.1 mg.

## Copper

Liver, kidney, nuts and raisins are rich sources of copper. Ninety-five percent of serum copper is present as ceruloplasmin. The latter is reduced or absent in the serum in Wilson's disease (hepatolenticular degeneration) and copper is deposited in the tissues (p. 181). It is believed that copper deficiency in children may cause neutropenia and the characteristic red depigmented hair occurring in kwashiorkor (p. 116).

## Fluorine

The effectiveness of fluorine in producing decay-resistant teeth is well-known. When the level of fluorine in drinking water exceeds 1 part per million (1 ppm), mottled enamel (fluorosis) occurs; the dentine is not affected.

Fluorides in soluble salts and in solution are absorbed almost completely from the gastrointestinal tract. In contrast the slowly soluble forms of fluoride such as those in calcium fluoride in bone meal are absorbed less readily and to a variable degree. Fluoride ion is in part excreted by the kidneys and in part stored in bone or developing teeth. Within physiologic limits the level of fluoride is kept as low as possible in the internal environment of the body.

Fluoride ion can replace hydroxyl (and perhaps carbonate) ions on the surface of apatite crystals in bone and substitute for hydroxyl ion in the formation of new bone. There is no danger to bone from the lifetime ingestion of fluoride from drinking water containing 1 ppm fluoride. It has been shown in one survey that only 23 patients from a total of 170,000 roentgen examinations of the spine and pelvis had increased density of bone resulting from the long-term use of drinking water containing 4 to 8 ppm of fluoride (Stevenson and Watson, 1957). In another survey it was found that the prevalence of osteoporosis and collapsed vertebrae in older people, especially women, was significantly less in communities using 4 to 8 ppm fluoride in the water supply than in those having 0.15 to 0.3 ppm fluoride (Bernstein et al., 1966).

In the teeth, the highest concentration of fluoride was found in the outer surface of the enamel (Brudevold et al., 1956). During the preeruptive period after calcification is completed fluoride deposition continues in the external surface and to a lesser extent after eruption.

## TRACE ELEMENTS

The trace elements chromium, cobalt, manganese, molybdenum, selenium and zinc are essential requirements for some animals and it is likely that they are also for man. Vitamin $B_{12}$ which is an essential dietary component for man contains cobalt (p. 121). Manganese is needed for normal bone structure and is a part of enzyme systems that occur in man.

These trace elements are found in green leafy foods, fruit, whole grains and meat and the risk of a deficiency is slight for the patient who eats a mixed diet.

## GENERAL REFERENCES

*Accepted Dental Therapeutics*, 33rd ed., Chicago, American Dental Association, 1970.
Diet and Nutrition: Practitioner, *201*, August, 1968.

Vitamin E
Majaj, A. S., Dinning, J. S., Azzam, S. A., and Darby, W. J.: Vitamin E responsive megaloblastic anemia in infants with protein-calorie malnutrition. Amer. J. Clin. Nutr., *12*, 374, 1963.

Fluorine
Bernstein, D. S., Sadowsky, N., and Hegsted, D. M.: Prevalence of osteoporosis in high- and low-fluoride areas in North Dakota. J.A.M.A., *198*, 499, 1966.
Brudevold, F., Gardner, D. E., and Smith, F A.: Distribution of fluoride in human enamel. J. Dent., Res. *35*, 420, 1956.
Stevenson, C. A. and Watson, R.: Fluoride osteosclerosis. Amer. J Roentgen., *78*, 13, 1957.

## SUGGESTED READING

*Fluid and Electrolytes*. Some practical guides to clinical use. Chicago, Abbott Laboratories, September, 1970.

## Chapter 11

# ENDOCRINE DISORDERS

The endocrine glands synthesize hormones and release them into the bloodstream. The mode of action of hormones, however, is poorly understood. It is known that some of the glands are dependent on and controlled by a specific hormone produced by the anterior pituitary. A lowering of the blood level of thyroid hormone will, for example, cause the thyroid-stimulating hormone (TSH) of the pituitary to be secreted and cause a rise in thyroid hormone. When the latter rises sufficiently, the secretion of a thyroid-stimulating hormone will cease. This is known as a "negative feed-back." The pituitary gland itself is controlled by the hypothalamus.

In the case of the parathyroids, secretion of parathyroid hormone is dependent on a low blood calcium level. When the blood calcium rises, the hormone secretion is suppressed.

Endocrine disease may be caused either by excess or deficiency of hormone. Excess of the hormone may be due to hyperplasia or tumor (which may be benign or malignant). Deficiency of hormone is due usually to atrophy or removal of the gland or infiltration by tumor or inflammatory or granulomatous tissue.

## PITUITARY

Hyperfunction of the eosinophil cells of the anterior pituitary results in gigantism or acromegaly depending on the time of onset. Dwarfism due to hypofunction of the eosinophil cells before puberty is rare. After puberty, hypofunction of the anterior pituitary may occur from pressure of a pituitary tumor and from postpartum pituitary necrosis (Sheehan's syndrome): the result is atrophy of the thyroid, adrenals and gonads.

Damage to the neurohypophysis may occur following severe head injury and may result in diabetes insipidus. This disease, which is uncommon, is caused by a deficiency of vasopressin (antidiuretic hormone, ADH); it is characterized by the excretion of large quantities of urine (polyuria) and increased thirst (polydipsia).

## Gigantism

This condition occurs if hyperfunction of the eosinophil cell occurs before closure of the epiphyses; if they are already closed, then acromegaly results. Gigantism is defined as a height exceeding 80 inches; the increase in size is due to disproportionately long arms and legs. When due to a pathologic process there is usually associated muscular weakness and the secondary sexual characteristics are poorly developed.

## Acromegaly

The signs and symptoms of acromegaly occur insidiously over a number of years. There is gradual enlargement of the hands and feet and coarsening of the facial features. The frontal sinuses increase in size, the mandible becomes enlarged, the tongue thickens and there is spacing of the teeth and alteration of the occlusion. The facial skin coarsens and there is enlargement of the nose and lips (Figure 11.1). Other early symptoms are head-

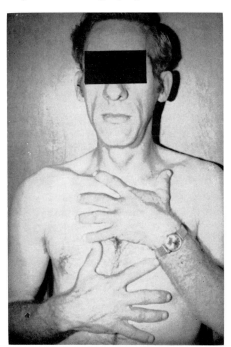

**Figure 11.1.** Acromegaly. There is coarsening of the facial features and increase in size of the hands. Male, aged 40 years. (*Courtesy of Dr. Gerald A. Williams*)

ache, tingling in the fingers, muscle pains and loss of libido.  Increase in the size of the larynx will produce deepening of the voice.  Pressure of the tumor on the optic chiasma will result in bitemporal hemianopsia in a proportion of cases.  Diabetes mellitus is present in up to 40 percent of cases.

DIAGNOSIS.  In both gigantism and acromegaly, a radiograph of the skull reveals resorption and increase in size of the sella turcica, usually with destruction of the clinoid processes.  In the active phase of acromegaly, the inorganic serum phosphate may be $> 4$ mg./100 ml.

TREATMENT.  Both syndromes can be treated by radiotherapy of the pituitary or by surgical removal of the tumor.

# THYROID

## Thyroid Hormones

The thyroid follicles manufacture two thyroid hormones, triiodothyronine ($T_3$) and thyroxine (tetraiodothyronine, $T_4$) which are released into the blood.  They exert a controlling influence on growth and metabolism.  The secretion of the thyroid hormones is controlled by thyroid stimulating hormones (TSH or thyrotropin) from the anterior pituitary gland.

The hormones released from the thyroid gland are rapidly bound to plasma proteins and only a small proportion of thyroxine and triiodothyronine are present in the free or active form.

### Calcitonin

This is a hormone found in the thyroid which inhibits bone resorption thus opposing the effect of parathyroid hormone on bone.

## Diseases of the Thyroid Gland

Diseases of the thyroid gland can be classified as:
1. Hyperthyroidism—thyrotoxicosis
2. Hypothyroidism—cretinism; myxedema
3. Goiter—endemic; multinodular
4. Thyroiditis—acute; chronic
5. Carcinoma

A goiter is an enlargement of the thyroid gland.  In the past, the term has been used to describe a number of thyroid enlargements but its use should be restricted to group 3 in the above classification.

### THYROID-FUNCTION TESTS

The following tests are used in the diagnosis of thyroid disease.

### Protein-bound Iodine (PBI)

The PBI test measures the level of circulating thyroid hormone by precipitating serum proteins and measuring their iodine content.  It also measures the iodides from medication and incomplete or abnormal iodine-bearing proteins such as iodinated tyrosines formed in thyroiditis or in certain enzyme deficiencies of the thyroid where hormone synthesis is defective. The PBI is increased in pregnancy or in patients taking the contraceptive pill and is decreased in patients who are taking salicylates or dilantin. The normal range is 4 to 8 $\mu$g. per 100 ml.

### Butanol-extractable Iodine (BEI)

This is a modified PBI test which measures iodine bound to protein in serum extracted with butanol. Although it excludes interfering iodides it measures x-ray contrast media which contain iodine. The normal range is 3 to 7 $\mu$g. per 100 ml.

### Serum Thyroxine (T₄)

Serum thyroxine can be measured by column chromatography and by competitive protein binding. The latter excludes both organic and inorganic iodides but medications such as antithyroid drugs, sex hormones and salicylates interfere with the results. The normal range of serum thyroxine by either method is 2.9 to 6.4 $\mu$g. per 100 ml.

### Free Thyroxine Concentration (Free T₄)

Free $T_4$ measures the very small amount of thyroxine which is not bound to plasma proteins. This test is not affected by any of the medications mentioned above. The normal range is 1 to 2.1 $\mu\mu$g. per 100 ml.

### T₃ Resin Uptake

Labelled triiodothyronine is added to serum and binds to sites on the binding protein not occupied by thyroid hormone. A resin is then added to the serum and absorbs all the unbound $T_3$. The results are altered by medications affecting binding such as sex hormones, diphenylhydantoin and salicylates. A high level indicates hyperthyroidism and a low level hypothyroidism. The normal range is 25 to 35 percent.

### Radioactive Iodine Uptake

The patient swallows a tracer dose of I[131] (half-life of eight days) and after a number of hours a count is made of the radioactivity absorbed by the gland. This is expressed as a percentage of total administered radioactivity. The radioactive iodine uptake is increased in hyperthyroidism and decreased in hypothyroidism. The normal uptake by the thyroid gland is 15 to 45 percent of the tracer dose in 24 hours.

### Basal Metabolic Rate (B.M.R.)

This is now used infrequently as it requires full cooperation of the patient which is not obtained easily if the patient is anxious, aged or slow mentally.

## Reflex Timing

The ankle reflex is timed using special instruments. The tendon reflex action is slow in hypothyroidism and fast in hyperthyroidism.

## Tanned Red Cell Agglutination Test

This test is used to determine autoimmunity against thyroid antigens.

## HYPERTHYROIDISM

### Thyrotoxicosis

ETIOLOGY. Although the cause of thyrotoxicosis is uncertain, there is in the sera of many thyrotoxic patients an autoantibody—LATS (long-acting thyroid stimulator)—which stimulates the release of thyroid hormone.

CLINICAL FEATURES. The common complaints are increased nervousness, sweating, loss of weight, intolerance of hot weather and diarrhea.

SIGNS. The eyes may be staring or obviously protruded. When the patient looks down the upper lid may lag behind the globe leaving a rim of sclera above the cornea, the so-called "lid lag" (Figure 11.2). There is frequently a fine tremor of the outstretched fingers. The pulse is rapid and in approximately 10 percent of patients, atrial fibrillation is present and may lead to heart failure. The thyrotoxic patient is usually thin with moist sweating palms.

The enlarged thyroid gland moves on swallowing and may be diffusely enlarged and soft or irregularly nodular and firm.

SPECIAL INVESTIGATIONS. The B.M.R. is raised and the plasma bound iodine is raised. The uptake of $I^{131}$ by the gland is increased and the serum cholesterol is reduced. The latter test may not always be reliable in hyperthyroidism.

TREATMENT. Antithyroid drugs may be given or $I^{131}$ may be used which is concentrated in the gland and destroys the thyroid tissue by radiation or the gland may be surgically removed. Some authorities restrict the use of radioactive iodine to patients over 40 years of age because of fear of inducing thyroid cancer.

DENTAL MANAGEMENT OF HYPERTHYROIDISM. The hyperthyroid patient is a poor candidate for routine dental treatment unless he is adequately sedated. Hyperthyroid individuals are particularly susceptible to untoward responses after epinephrine.

## HYPOTHYROIDISM

### Cretinism

This condition, which occurs in infants and young children, results from a deficiency of thyroid hormones during fetal or early life. In cretins, the thyroid may be congenitally absent or greatly reduced in size and its sub-

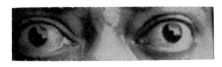

**Figure 11.2.** Thyrotoxicosis. Despite the pronounced exophthalmos the thyroid gland was not markedly enlarged. Male, aged 35 years. (*Courtesy of Dr. Gerald A. Williams*)

stance replaced by fibrous tissue or lymphocytes. As a result, the child's entire physical and mental development is retarded.

CLINICAL FEATURES. The child has a thick skin which later becomes dry, wrinkled and sallow. The tongue is enlarged, lips thickened, mouth open and drooling. The face is broad and the nose is flattened. Umbilical hernia and enlargement of the abdomen usually develop. The infant is dull and apathetic, usually constipated and has a subnormal temperature. The child is mentally retarded. The eruption of teeth is delayed.

TREATMENT. Thyroid extract or sodium levothyroxine.

## Myxedema

This condition which occurs in the adult may result from surgical excision or from primary atrophy of the gland or may develop secondary to hypofunction of the anterior lobe of the pituitary.

CLINICAL FEATURES. The patient has the characteristic non-pitting subcutaneous swelling seen particularly on the face as a puffiness around the eyes. There is loss of the lateral third of the eyebrows. The tongue is large and the speech is slow and deep-toned. Mental apathy, drowsiness and sensitivity to cold are common. A slow relaxation of the tendon reflexes is often present.

SPECIAL INVESTIGATIONS. The B.M.R., $I^{131}$ uptake and PBI are all low, whereas the serum cholesterol is often high. There is usually an iron-deficiency anemia.

TREATMENT. Desiccated thyroid or sodium levothyroxine must be given throughout life.

## GOITER

### Endemic Goiter

This is a diffuse, soft, symmetric enlargement of the gland without hyperthyroidism. It is caused by lack of iodine and tends to occur in those areas in which the soil and water lack iodine but it may also result from a genetic failure of enzymes. It can be prevented by the use of iodized table salt.

### Multinodular Goiter

This condition is encountered most frequently in patients over age 30. The gland contains rounded swellings of varying size. Complications are:

1. Pressure upon the trachea
2. Secondary thyrotoxicosis
3. Carcinoma—carcinomatous change occurs in about eight percent of cases.

TREATMENT. Subtotal thyroidectomy to prevent the previously mentioned complications.

## THYROIDITIS

### Acute Thyroiditis

Acute thyroiditis is usually preceded by an upper respiratory infection. The inflammation of the gland may progress to suppuration and abscess formation. The onset is acute and the gland is red, swollen and tender.

TREATMENT. Cultures are taken and the appropriate antibiotic is administered.

### Chronic Thyroiditis

There are two varieties of this condition, both of unknown origin, developing gradually in young to middle-aged women without previous history of trauma or infection. The common type is *Hashimoto's disease* (lymphadenoid goiter) which is characterized by moderate enlargement of the gland with a firm, smooth or lobular surface and is believed to be an autoimmune disorder. Histologic examination shows extensive lymphoid infiltration. The second type, *Riedel's struma*, is very rare and is characterized by an enlarged gland which is hard and adherent to adjacent structures but not to the skin. Histologically, there is extensive fibrosis with atrophic follicles.

TREATMENT. If left untreated, both types proceed to myxedema. Subtotal thyroidectomy followed by oral thyroid is the treatment of choice.

## CARCINOMA

Carcinomata of the thyroid may be subdivided histologically into several types ranging from an extremely anaplastic tumor to a well-differentiated adenocarcinoma. These conditions are described in textbooks of surgery.

## PARATHYROID

### Hyperparathyroidism

ETIOLOGY. The disease is due to excess secretion of parathyroid hormone usually by an adenoma or, less commonly, by hyperplasia of the parathyroid glands resulting in elevation of the blood calcium. Calcium is removed from the bones giving rise to skeletal disease and is excreted via the kidneys resulting in renal stones.

CLINICAL FEATURES. The hypercalcemia may produce muscular weakness, anorexia, constipation, polyuria and thirst. The bone disease presents as bone pain, pathologic fractures, and the "brown tumor" of hyperparathyroidism which in the jaws may resemble a giant cell reparative granuloma. The radiographic findings may include generalized bone rarefaction, multiple radiolucent areas, subperiosteal bone resorption of terminal phalanges and loss of lamina dura of the teeth.

Renal calculi are a common manifestation and renal colic may be the presenting symptom.

LABORATORY TESTS. The serum calcium is usually $> 11$ mg./100 ml. and the serum phosphate is low. Serum alkaline phosphatase may be increased especially in the presence of significant bone disease.

TREATMENT. Surgical removal of the adenoma or, if diffuse parathyroid hyperplasia is discovered, subtotal parathyroidectomy should be performed.

### Hypoparathyroidism

ETIOLOGY. Hypoparathyroidism usually follows accidental removal of or damage to the parathyroid glands during thyroidectomy. Because of the deficiency of parathyroid hormone, there is a low serum calcium and a high serum phosphate level and the patient has a tendency to develop tetany.

CLINICAL FEATURES. In the latent stages of tetany, signs of increased neuromuscular excitability may be elicited. The two most important signs are *Chvostek's sign* which is spasm of the facial muscles produced by tapping the facial nerve just in front of the ear and *Trousseau's sign* which is spasm of the hand following temporary occlusion of the blood supply in the arm. One of the first symptoms may be a circumoral paresthesia and tonic contractions may occur spontaneously. These most frequently involve the muscles of the hands and feet, face, eyes, tongue and larynx. When the larynx is involved, laryngeal stridor occurs and tracheostomy may be necessary.

LABORATORY TESTS. The serum calcium is low, the serum phosphate is high, alkaline phosphatase may be normal or low and there is absence of urinary calcium.

TREATMENT. Calcium gluconate, calcium lactate and large doses of vitamin D.

### ADRENAL

The adrenal gland consists of the cortex and medulla. The medulla secretes epinephrine and norepinephrine and the cortex, which is essential to life, secretes a number of steroid hormones. The hormones produced by the adrenal cortex are referred to as corticosteroids or adrenocortical hormones. Of these hormones, cortisol and aldosterone are essential for life. The corticosteroids are important in the regulation of protein, fat and carbohydrate metabolism and salt and water balance.

## ADRENOCORTICOTROPHIC HORMONE (ACTH)

ACTH is produced by the basophil and chromophobe cells of the pituitary gland and causes the release of steroid hormones by the adrenal glands. The release of ACTH is effected by the corticotrophin-releasing factor (CRF) which is produced in the hypothalamus and travels in the pituitary stalk portal blood to the anterior pituitary gland. The principal regulatory mechanism for CRF release is the level of free cortisol in the plasma. When plasma cortisol is low there is an increased release of CRF and when plasma cortisol concentration is elevated, there is a decreased release of CRF.

## The Adrenal Cortex

### HORMONES OF THE ADRENAL CORTEX

Although a number of adrenal steroid hormones have been isolated from the adrenal cortex, the main ones found in adrenal vein blood are cortisol, corticosterone, aldosterone, dehydroepiandrosterone (DHA), △4-androstenedione and 11β-hydroxyandrostenedione. Each day the human adrenal secretes about 25 mg. of cortisol, 2 mg. of corticosterone, 200 μg. of aldosterone and 25 mg. of DHA.

It is convenient to group these hormones into three types according to their main metabolic activities:

1. *Glucocorticoids*, principally cortisol (hydrocortisone).
2. *Mineralocorticoids*, aldosterone, 11-deoxycorticosterone and corticosterone. Aldosterone is the principal mineralocorticoid.
3. *Androgens*, DHA, △4-androstenedione and 11β-hydroxyandrostenedione.

The division of adrenal steroids into glucocorticoids and mineralocorticoids is somewhat arbitrary in that most glucocorticoids have some mineralocorticoid-like activity and vice versa. Corticosteroids, a term which includes glucocorticoids and mineralocorticoids, are $C_{21}$ compounds which implies a molecule with 21 carbon atoms.

### Glucocorticoids (Cortisol)

The glucocorticoids promote the formation of glucose from the breakdown of protein (gluconeogenesis), stimulate fat deposition especially over the abdomen and between the scapulae, increase muscle strength and efficiency, increase renal blood flow and reduce the intensity of the inflammatory reaction.

### Mineralocorticoids (Aldosterone, 11-Deoxycorticosterone, Corticosterone)

The mineralocorticoids increase reabsorption of sodium by the renal tubule and promote excretion of potassium in the urine. In excess they may produce hypertension, hypokalemia (low potassium) and alkalosis. The secretion of aldosterone is believed to be controlled by angiotensin II (see p. 57).

### Adrenal Androgens (Dehydroepiandrosterone, △4-Androstenedione, 11β-Hydroxyandrostenedione)

The androgens cause masculinization including enlargement of the larynx, increased body and facial hair, balding in the temporal regions, increased muscle mass and positive nitrogen balance. In the female androgens will in addition produce amenorrhea, atrophy of the breasts and uterus, and enlargement of the clitoris; in the male the sexual organs enlarge.

The androgens are metabolized in the liver and excreted in the urine. Two-thirds of the urine 17-ketosteroids in the male are derived from adrenal metabolites, and the remaining one-third comes from testicular secretion of testosterone. In the female almost all the urine 17-ketosteroids are derived exclusively from adrenal gland secretions.

The androgens, which contain 19 carbon atoms, have an oxygen atom at C-17, hence their designation 17-ketosteroids.

## METABOLISM OF THE CORTICOSTEROIDS

Some steroids, such as cortisol, are reduced in the liver and then excreted in the urine. Others are conjugated with glucuronic acid and then excreted in the urine.

## TESTS OF ADRENAL CORTICAL FUNCTION

### Blood Levels

The blood levels of ACTH, cortisol and aldosterone can be measured.

### Urine Levels

Tests are available which enable the urine levels of 17-hydroxycorticoids, 17-ketosteroids and 17-ketogenic steroids to be estimated.

17-HYDROXYCORTICOIDS. Cortisol, cortisone (a synthetic steroid) and their tetrahydro metabolites which have a hydroxyl group at $C_{17}$ react with phenylhydrazine to give a yellow color, and are referred to as 17-hydroxycorticoids or 17-hydroxycorticosteroids. (This is the Porter-Silber reaction, and these steroids are often called Porter-Silber chromogens.) The method can be applied to urine or to blood. For most clinical purposes, the determination of the 24-hour urinary excretion of total 17-hydroxycorticoids provides a satisfactory measurement of adrenocortical function and one which is more specific than the 17-ketosteroid determination, particularly in the male. The normal adult resting values range from one to ten mg. in 24 hours.

17-KETOSTEROIDS. The term "17-ketosteroids" refers to steroids having a ketone group on the $C_{17}$ of the steroid nucleus. 17-Ketosteroids may be derived from androgens originating in the adrenal cortex and testis.

In the female, the 17-ketosteroids are primarily of adrenal origin. Whereas in the male approximately one-third are of testicular origin, the remainder coming from the adrenal cortex.

The urinary 17-ketosteroids are determined by the Zimmerman reaction. The normal values range from 7 to 25 mg. per 24 hours for adult men and from 5 to 15 mg. for women. Lower values are found in children.

17-KETOGENIC STEROIDS. The method employed depends on the fact

10

that $C_{21}$ adrenocortical hormones (glucocorticoids and mineralocorticoids) can be oxidized to 17-ketosteroids and then determined by the Zimmerman reaction (see above). In both men and women, normal excretion of 17-ketogenic steroids is 5 to 20 mg. in 24 hours. The original urinary 17-ketosteroids must be either inactivated or measured separately before the 17-ketogenic steroids are studied.

## Stimulation Tests

It is important to distinguish primary adrenal failure from that secondary to failure of the pituitary to secrete ACTH.

ACTH is given intravenously on two successive days and the complete 24-hour urine output is analyzed for steroid levels. Normally, there is an increase in the urinary steroids. If there is no increase, this indicates that the adrenal glands are not functioning normally.

## Suppression Tests

If dexamethasone, a potent glucocorticoid, is administered to a normal individual on two successive days, there is a reduction in ACTH produced by the pituitary and a fall in the urine 17-hydroxycorticoid level. A normal response to this suppression implies that the adrenal glands are under the control of ACTH.

## Metyrapone (Metopirone) Test

The metyrapone test is used for evaluation of the reserve capacity of the anterior pituitary to release ACTH. Metyrapone is a drug that interferes with the conversion of 11-deoxycortisol (Compound S) to cortisol. Because 11-deoxycortisol is a weak suppressor of the feedback mechanism causing release of ACTH, the anterior pituitary responds by releasing larger quantities of ACTH in an attempt to stimulate the adrenal gland to release additional cortisol. This, however, is prevented because of the block induced by metyrapone. The normal individual responds to this test with at least a doubling of their basal 17-hydroxycorticoid excretion.

## DISEASES OF THE ADRENAL CORTEX

There are a number of clinical syndromes associated with excessive secretion of the adrenal cortical hormones. Excess production of cortisol is associated with Cushing's syndrome; excess production of aldosterone with aldosteronism; excess production of adrenal androgens with adrenal virilism. These syndromes on occasion tend to overlap. Adrenal insufficiency results in Addison's disease.

## Cushing's Syndrome

This syndrome is most commonly associated with adrenal hyperplasia. Other less common causes are prolonged treatment with glucocorticoids and ACTH, ACTH-producing tumors of the pituitary, and benign and malignant tumors of the adrenal.

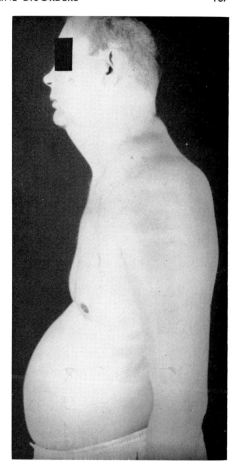

**Figure 11.3.** Cushing's syndrome. Associated with adrenal hyperplasia. Note the 'moon face', 'buffalo hump' and obesity of the trunk. Male, aged 42 years. (*Courtesy of Dr. Gerald A. Williams*)

CLINICAL FEATURES. This syndrome is three times more common in the female than in the male. The face is plethoric and round ('moon' face), there is obesity of the trunk and interscapular fat deposition resulting in the so-called 'buffalo hump' (Figure 11.3). In addition, hypertension, weakness, amenorrhea, hirsutism, purplish striae over the abdomen, edema, glycosuria, and osteoporosis may be present. As stated previously the glucocorticoids cause increased protein breakdown: loss of protein from the dermis causes the vessels to shine through the skin and because their support is lost easy bruising occurs. Loss of protein from the vertebrae results in osteoporosis and in some cases fractures occur.

LABORATORY FINDINGS. There is increased cortisol production which can be measured in the blood. The 17-hydroxycorticoids are elevated in severe cases. Most patients with this syndrome have glucosuria and some have frank diabetes necessitating insulin therapy.

TREATMENT. When due to adrenal tumor or hyperplasia surgery is indicated. When due to pituitary tumor, hypophysectomy or implantation of yttrium[90] pellets into the pituitary are employed.

### Adrenal Insufficiency (Addison's Disease)

ETIOLOGY. The most common cause of the disease is destruction of the gland by tuberculosis followed by idiopathic atrophy.

SYMPTOMS AND SIGNS. Weakness and easy fatigability are early symptoms. There is increased pigmentation of the skin especially at pressure points and of the mucous membranes. Typically, melanin pigmentation occurs anywhere in the oral cavity but commonly on the buccal mucosa. Weight loss, dehydration, and a low blood pressure are characteristic. Anorexia, nausea, vomiting and diarrhea often occur.

LABORATORY TESTS. The lack of aldosterone results in reduced serum levels of sodium and chloride with increase of potassium.

TREATMENT. Replacement therapy with cortisone and fludrocortisone, a synthetic mineralocorticoid, is employed.

### The Adrenal Medulla

The adrenal medulla synthesizes the catecholamines—epinephrine and norepinephrine—from the amino acid tyrosine.

## ACTIONS OF THE CATECHOLAMINES

Epinephrine produces the following effects:
1. Raises the blood glucose by promoting glycogenolysis in the liver and muscles
2. Increases the basal metabolic rate
3. Produces the sensations of excitement and fear
4. Increases the cardiac output
5. Raises the plasma free fatty acids from neutral fat depots

Norepinephrine produces the following effects:
1. Raises the blood pressure by constricting peripheral vessels
2. Raises the plasma free fatty acids by stimulating lipolysis in adipose tissue

Norepinephrine has only slight effects on the blood glucose, central nervous system and metabolic rate.

## PHEOCHROMOCYTOMA

This is a rare tumor of the adrenal medulla the adverse effects of which are related to the continuous or intermittent secretion of epinephrine and norepinephrine.

CLINICAL FEATURES. The condition occurs in either sex usually between the ages of 25 and 55 years. Hypertension is associated with headaches, sweating, palpitations, tremor and hyperglycemia. Direct estimations of catecholamines or their degradation products in blood and urine are made to establish the diagnosis. An intravenous injection of phentolamine

(Regitine) will produce a fall of more than 25 mms. Hg in the diastolic pressure in a patient with a pheochromocytoma. Currently, this test is being replaced by quantitative estimation of urinary catecholamines or their metabolites, e.g., vanillylmandelic acid.

TREATMENT is excision of the tumor.

## THE PANCREAS

### Diabetes Mellitus

Diabetes mellitus is a disease in which there is reduced activity of insulin with resulting impaired carbohydrate tolerance. Some patients may have a family history of the disease.

PATHOLOGY. The primary pathologic change in diabetes is found in the islets of Langerhans of the pancreas. It is now believed that there is a correlation between the severity of diabetes and a reduction in the number of beta cells together with the degree of beta cell degranulation. Later in the disease hyaline degeneration, fibrosis and atrophy are the most frequent findings. Thickening of the basement membrane of the small arterioles is found in most parts of the body but important clinical effects are produced in the kidneys, retina, nervous system and skin.

BIOCHEMICAL CHANGES. Insulin is necessary for the active transport of glucose across the cell membrane. In diabetes, glucose enters the cells with difficulty so that its utilization by the tissues is impaired. Normally, insulin increases the storage of glycogen in the liver but in diabetes the liver is unable satisfactorily to convert glucose to glycogen. The blood glucose level rises and glucose begins to enter the renal tubules so rapidly that it cannot be reabsorbed, consequently glycosuria develops. Because of the failure of glucose to enter the adipose tissue cells, fat is mobilized as a source of energy and produces a rise in the free fatty acids and triglycerides of the plasma and of the triglycerides in the liver. The reduced availability of glucose results in the utilization of fatty acids which are converted into ketone bodies (acetone, acetoacetic acid and $\beta$-hydroxybutyric acid) and appear in the blood and urine.

The effects of the ketosis, partly due to the associated diuresis from glucosuria include negative balances of water, sodium, chloride, potassium and nitrogen. The ketones produce a 'metabolic acidosis' with a fall in blood pH and an associated fall in total blood bicarbonate ion.

In diabetes if there is marked inhibition of carbohydrate metabolism, protein breakdown is increased and wasting occurs.

CLINICAL FEATURES. The disease is characterized by hyperglycemia, glycosuria, polydipsia, hunger, pruritus, weakness and weight loss.

It is usual to separate the disease into "juvenile" and "maturity-onset" types. In the "juvenile" type there is more time available for complications to arise whereas in the "maturity-onset" type complications are less frequent.

In children or young adults, the onset may be abrupt but in older patients the disease is usually more insidious and may be discovered on routine urine examination. The older patients are frequently obese, ketosis is uncommon and the disorder can frequently be treated by dietary restrictions alone.

Some patients may have latent diabetes by which it is meant that no signs or symptoms of the disease are present but there is an abnormal glucose tolerance test or an elevated fasting blood glucose when not under stress. Women with latent diabetes may bear abnormally heavy children and in later life may manifest overt diabetes.

ORAL MANIFESTATIONS. Because of the lowered resistance to infections in diabetes, the diabetic is prone to develop severe periodontal disease and apical infections. Dryness of the mouth is an early manifestation.

LABORATORY FINDINGS. If the fasting venous blood sugar is $> 110$ mg./100 ml. or the blood sugar two hours after a meal is $> 120$ mg./100 ml. diabetes mellitus is the presumptive diagnosis. To confirm the diagnosis a glucose tolerance test is required.

TREATMENT. In the obese diabetic whose diabetes commences after middle-age, diet alone may suffice or hypoglycemic drugs may be prescribed. The younger diabetic requires insulin by injection and a regulated diet.

## COURSE AND COMPLICATIONS

In young diabetics, blood vessel involvement is common later in life. Coronary disease may produce angina pectoris or coronary occlusion. There may be decreased arterial supply to the limbs resulting in intermittent claudication and gangrene. In addition degenerative changes may occur in the small blood vessels of the retina and result in failing vision.

The diabetic is prone to skin infections, such as recurrent furuncles and carbuncles. Pulmonary tuberculosis is about twice as common in diabetics as non-diabetics.

### Diabetic Neuropathy

Nerve lesions occur in diabetics and may be cranial or peripheral. The sixth cranial nerve is most frequently affected resulting in lateral rectus palsy. Involvement of peripheral motor nerves may manifest as weakness of muscles. Sensory nerve involvement may cause a variety of symptoms ranging from paresthesias to severe pain.

### Diabetic Coma

This is the result of ketosis and may be the first manifestation of the disease. In the diabetic who is receiving insulin it may occur because of inadequate insulin dosage or an infection which reduces the effectiveness of insulin. The patient is drowsy or comatose and dehydrated. The skin is hot and dry and the eyes are soft and shrunken with dilated pupils. The blood pressure is low and the pulse is fast. The respiration is deep and there is a smell of acetone in the breath. The treatment is discussed below under oral surgery in the diabetic.

## Insulin Reactions (Hypoglycemia)

Overdosage with insulin or failure to eat a meal after an insulin injection will result in a fall of blood sugar to 40 mg./100 ml. or lower. Hypoglycemia results in a massive outpouring of epinephrine and the result is tachycardia, anxiety, sweating, pallor and rise of blood pressure. Nervous system abnormalities may occur which take the form of confusion, hallucinations, hyperactivity, convulsions and finally coma. If the patient is conscious sugar may be given by mouth, otherwise intravenous glucose is necessary.

## ORAL SURGERY IN THE DIABETIC

A surgical operation in a diabetic may well upset the control of his diabetes because of the effect of the anesthesia, the surgical trauma, the nutritional and fluid balance and the altered physical activity.

Before the diabetic patient is admitted for oral surgery, it is important to consult with his physician concerning his general health, the daily dose of insulin, the type of insulin used or, if the patient is taking an oral hypoglycemic agent, the daily dose of the particular drug. The laboratory procedures performed routinely on admission are a complete blood count, urinalysis, blood tests for glucose, blood urea nitrogen and electrolytes. In addition, an electrocardiogram and chest radiograph are required.

It is preferable to schedule the operation early in the morning so that if insulin is to be given it can be covered by a glucose infusion which replaces the carbohydrate usually taken at breakfast.

The management of the diabetic patient during oral surgery depends on whether the surgery is emergency or elective.

### Emergency Surgery

Under this heading can be considered the treatment of pulpally and periodontally involved teeth which are causing pain. Local analgesia is preferable but may not always be possible.

Diabetic patients who have previously been well-controlled may be admitted in diabetic coma as a result of an abscessed tooth or a pericoronal infection around an erupting mandibular third molar tooth. Vigorous treatment is initiated with five-percent dextrose in water administered intravenously and regular insulin is given intramuscularly. The object of the therapy is to correct ketosis and dehydration. Control of the patient is assessed every one to six hours by measuring urinary glucose, the blood acetone, $CO_2$, sugar and electrolytes. The infection is treated with the appropriate antibiotic by injection. When the patient begins to respond to the therapy an anesthetic can be administered and pus drained.

### Elective Surgery

Elective surgery may be defined as surgery for which the patient is admitted as a routine procedure.

The severity of diabetes is usually judged by the patient's history. Those who are controlled by diet alone or diet and oral hypoglycemic agents may be considered mild diabetics. These patients are usually able to withstand the stress of most elective surgical procedures with little or no change in blood sugar. When glycosuria and hyperglycemia occur, regular insulin is indicated in preference to the oral hypoglycemic agent.

A moderate diabetic is a patient who is satisfactorily controlled with one or two daily doses of intermediate-acting insulin either alone or in combination with short-acting insulin.

A severe or 'brittle' diabetic is a patient who is prone to ketosis and who experiences hypoglycemia with only slight overdosage of insulin.

In the management of the insulin-dependent patient undergoing surgery half the usual dosage of medium-acting or long-acting insulin is given before the patient is taken to the operating room. An intravenous infusion of 1000 ml. of five-percent dextrose in water is started immediately. The other half of the usual dosage of insulin is given in the recovery room. Insulin should not be added to the infusion as part of it is lost by absorption to the infusion bottle and tubing.

Additional amounts of glucose in water (usually 500 to 1000 ml.) are given postoperatively if oral feedings are contraindicated or not tolerated. A blood sugar determination should be made routinely several hours after completion of surgery as a check against insulin overdosage or underdosage. It is usually found that no more insulin is required until the next morning when the usual dose schedule may be resumed.

## THE OVARY

The ovary secretes estrogens, progesterone and androgens. The biosynthesis of the ovarian hormones is dependent on the pituitary gonadotropins and is normally cyclic, unless fertilization of an ovum occurs, in which cases ovarian secretion becomes continuous.

### Estrogens

Estradiol-17$\beta$ is the principal estrogen secreted and is the most potent. In the liver it is partly degraded to less potent estrogens, principally estrone and estriol. All three estrogens circulate in the blood bound to protein. They are conjugated in the liver with glucuronic and sulphuric acids and excreted in the bile and in the urine.

### ACTIONS OF ESTROGENS

The principal local effects are on the female genitalia. Estrogens cause the proliferation of the endometrium during the first half of the menstrual cycle. The thickness of the uterine muscle and the cornification of the vaginal epithelium are also dependent upon estrogens. In addition, estrogens are responsible for the female distribution of fat. Although estrogens stimulate growth, excessive levels may lead to short stature due to premature fusion of the epiphyses.

When large doses of estrogens are given to males, as in the treatment of carcinoma of the prostate, enlargement of the breasts and pigmentation of the nipples occur and there is testicular atrophy.

## Progesterone

Progesterone is secreted by the corpus luteum. In addition it is also synthesized in the adrenal cortex and testes. It is thought to circulate in the blood bound to protein and is excreted in the urine as the inactive conjugate pregnanediol glucuronide.

## ACTIONS OF PROGESTERONE

During the latter half of the menstrual cycle progesterone is responsible for the secretory changes in the endometrial glands. It also increases uterine motility and produces alveolar enlargement of the breast.

## Androgens

Under normal conditions, androgens, particularly androstenedione, are secreted in very small amounts by the ovary.

Androgen secretion is greatly increased in some pathologic conditions such as Stein-Leventhal syndrome (polycystic ovaries, infertility and hirsutism) and arrhenoblastoma, a rare tumor of the ovary.

## The Menopause

Usually in the late forties the secretion of estrogens and progesterone is diminished and ovulation ceases. The periods become more scanty and finally cease. Atrophic changes occur in the uterus, vagina and breasts and the pubic and axillary hair become more sparse. A feeling of warmth in the face, neck and upper chest associated with flushing (hot flashes) may occur at this time. These symptoms are thought to result from the combination of low estrogen and high gonadotropin levels. Nervousness, irritability and depression are not uncommon during the menopause. The hot flashes may be treated by administering estrogens three weeks in every month for three to six months.

## DENTAL IMPLICATIONS

Some postmenopausal patients may develop red, painful gingivae which bleed readily with minimal trauma. The condition, which is termed chronic desquamative gingivitis or gingivosis, may be associated with low estrogen levels in which case it will respond to estrogen therapy. It should be emphasized that not all cases of chronic desquamative gingivitis are the result of estrogen deficiency.

### The Effect of Pregnancy on the Teeth and Supporting Structures

Some females tend to have bleeding of the gingivae for the first time during pregnancy. This may be the result of local factors such as plaque or calculus or it may be the effect of hormones. The latter have been implicated in the genesis of pregnancy tumors. Neglected oral hygiene will result in dental caries, particularly around the gingival margins. Actual mobility of teeth may occur but following parturition the degree of mobility returns to normal.

### DENTAL RADIOGRAPHY DURING PREGNANCY

This should be avoided or kept to a minimum. If necessary, fast films, a collimator and a protective apron are used.

### ANESTHESIA DURING PREGNANCY

Local anesthesia is perfectly safe. During general anesthesia it is necessary to avoid hypotension as this may lead to placental separation. Similarly, hypoxia should be avoided.

## TESTIS

Between the seminiferous tubules of the testis in the adult lie small clumps of Leydig cells which produce the male sex hormones or androgens. In the child the Leydig cells are absent; they make their appearance just prior to puberty in response to interstitial cell stimulating hormone (ICSH) of the pituitary which is probably the same as luteinizing hormone (LH) in the female. Follicle stimulating hormone (FSH) of the pituitary is essential for the final stages of spermatogenesis after puberty.

### Testosterone

Testosterone is the most important testicular hormone and is carried in the plasma bound to protein. It is metabolized mainly in the liver and then conjugated with sulfates or glucuronic acid to be excreted in the urine as 17-ketosteroids, primarily androsterone and etiocholanolone. The testis contributes about 30 percent of the 17-ketosteroids in man, the remainder coming from the adrenal cortex.

### Testicular Androgens

Before puberty, excess androgen from a functioning testicular tumor will accelerate linear growth of the skeleton and cause precocious sexual development. At puberty testicular androgens cause enlargement of the larynx with deepening of the voice, increase in rate of linear growth and maturation of skeletal development leading to fusion of epiphyses. There is enlargement of the penis and scrotum. Hair grows on the face, axillae, chest, pubis and on the anterior abdominal wall and recession of hair occurs at the temples. An increase in libido and aggressive attitudes occur.

Androgens have an anabolic effect and cause retention of nitrogen, phosphorus and other minerals.

## CHROMOSOMAL ABNORMALITIES

Man has 46 chromosomes of which 22 pairs are autosomes and a single pair is sex chromosomes—XX in the female and XY in the male.

### Barr Body

This is a small basophilic chromatin mass adjacent to the inner aspect of the nuclear membrane and is found in the nuclei of the normal human female. Sex chromatin determinations are most frequently made on buccal smears and it is found that 30 to 50 percent of the cells possess Barr bodies. Cells possessing sex chromatin are called chromatin-positive and those without it are chromatin-negative.

Two syndromes are associated with abnormalities of the gonads in which an abnormal number of sex chromosomes occurs. These are Klinefelter's syndrome in which there is an excess of sex chromosomes and Turner's syndrome in which there is a reduction in the number of sex chromosomes.

### Klinefelter's Syndrome

This syndrome is found in men who have small testes, aspermia, gynecomastia (well-developed breasts), and long arms and legs. Their cells are chromatin-positive as in women and they have 47 chromosomes with XXY sex chromosomes.

### Turner's Syndrome

This condition occurs in women who are usually short in stature, have webbing of the neck and a shield-like chest with widely spaced nipples. Underdevelopment of the genitals is often found and the patient does not menstruate. Coarctation of the aorta is an anomaly often found with this syndrome. The cells are chromatin-negative as in man and there are 45 chromosomes with a single X chromosome.

### Hermaphroditism

In true hermaphroditism which is rare, there is a mingling of the sexual characteristics and genitalia of both sexes. Thus patients may either have XX or XY sex chromosomes and both male and female gonads.

## DOWN'S SYNDROME (MONGOLISM)

Although this syndrome is not an abnormality of the sex chromosomes, it is placed here for convenience. The disease is usually associated with 47 chromosomes in which there are 3 free 21 chromosomes (trisomy-21).

CLINICAL FEATURES. The syndrome is characterized by mental deficiency and a number of diagnostic features. There is a typical facies with a broad face, high cheek bones, small nose and eyes slanting upward and outward with prominent epicanthal folds. The fifth fingers are short and curve inwards and there is one major crease on both the palms and soles. The genitals are small. Muscular hypotonia and joint hypermobility are present. In a considerable number of cases, congenital cardiac defects are present. Respiratory infections are frequent. An interesting radiographic feature is that the sinuses are frequently found to be absent. In Down's syndrome the incidence of leukemia is significantly increased.

## GENERAL REFERENCES

Fletcher, R. F.: *Lecture Notes on Endocrinology*, Oxford, Blackwell Scientific Publications, 1967.

Hall, R., Anderson, J., and Smart, G. A.: *Clinical Endocrinology*, Philadelphia, Lippincott, 1969.

Paschkis, K. E., Rakoff, A. E., Cantarow, A., and Rupp, J. J.: *Clinical Endocrinology*, 3rd ed., New York, Hoeber, 1967.

DIABETES

Breidahl, H. D., Martin, F. I. R., Semple, B., Walpole, G. R., Shepherd, D. U., Proust, A. J., and Harcourt, D.: Diabetes mellitus: diagnosis and treatment. Med. J. Aust., *2*, 759, 1968.

Podolsky, S.: Special needs of the diabetic undergoing surgery. Postgrad. Med., *45*, 128, 1969.

Steinke, J.: Management of diabetes mellitus and surgery. New Eng. J. Med., *282*, 1472, 1970.

THYROID FUNCTION

Hamburger, J. I.: When and how to use newer thyroid-function tests. Consultant, *10*, 38, 1970.

Chapter 12

# DISEASES OF THE BONES AND JOINTS

Bone is composed of an organic matrix (osteoid) in which are deposited bone crystals consisting mainly of hydroxyapatite together with small amounts of other ions such as carbonate, citrate, sodium and magnesium. The osteoblasts, which connect with each other by cytoplasmic arms, secrete the organic intercellular substance of bone. When the osteoblasts are completely surrounded by the intercellular substance they have secreted, they are termed osteocytes. Bone is resorbed by osteoclasts, the number of which is increased by parathyroid hormone.

In growing bones, bone deposition exceeds bone resorption. When growth is over, these two processes are in balance. In old age bone resorption tends to exceed bone deposition and the bones become less dense. This condition is termed osteoporosis.

## DISEASES OF BONE

Bone may be involved by inflammations both acute and chronic, deficiency states, general diseases and tumors both benign and malignant. In addition, malignant tumors of breast, thyroid, prostate, adrenals, kidney and bronchus may metastasize to bone.

BONE BIOPSY. To confirm the diagnosis of a bone disease, a plug of bone is removed with a trephine from the iliac crest or from another affected bone. Some of the bone is decalcified, sectioned and stained; from the remainder, ground sections are prepared. If the biopsy is taken from an affected area of bone, a diagnosis can be made from the prepared section.

The diseases which will be considered here are:

1. Deficiency states
   a. Rickets
   b. Osteomalacia
   c. Osteoporosis
   d. Scurvy
2. General diseases of bone
   a. Osteogenesis imperfecta
   b. Cleidocranial dysostosis
   c. Osteopetrosis (Albers-Schönberg disease)
   d. Achondroplasia
   e. Infantile cortical hyperostosis (Caffey's disease)
   f. Paget's disease (osteitis deformans)
   g. Fibrous dysplasia of bone
   h. Leontiasis ossea
   i. Hyperparathyroidism

## Deficiency States

### RICKETS

Rickets is seen in children who have been fed a diet deficient in vitamin D. Good sources of this vitamin include liver, butter fat, egg yolk, fish-liver oil and fortified milk and margarine. Endogenous vitamin D is derived from a provitamin, 7-dehydrocholesterol, which is present in human epidermis. Exposure to the ultraviolet irradiation of the sun's rays converts 7-dehydrocholesterol into the active form, which is called vitamin $D_3$. Vitamin D promotes calcium absorption from the gut and mineral deposition in the skeleton.

In rickets, there is defective deposition of calcium salts in the cartilage matrix of the growing ends of the bones. Because of the defective mineralization, the bones soften and become deformed (Figure 12.1).

CLINICAL FEATURES. The skeletal deformities seen depend on the age of the child. In the infant who is recumbent, the effects of pressure produce flattening of the skull, thorax and pelvic girdle. If the child can walk, bowing of the long bones occurs and, in addition, vertebral and pelvic deformities may ensue. Beading of the costochondral junctions or rachitic rosary occurs and may be difficult to differentiate from similar changes which take place in scurvy. The sternum may be pushed forward resulting in the so-called "pigeon breast." The teeth may be delayed in erupting and, if the disease was operative during enamel calcification, enamel hypoplasia may result.

LABORATORY DIAGNOSIS. The serum calcium level is generally normal or at the lower limit of normal. Serum phosphorus values are reduced from the normal childhood level of 5 to 6 mg. to 2 to 4 mg. per 100 ml. The alkaline phosphatase level is generally elevated and remains so until weeks after therapy has been instituted.

TREATMENT is to administer vitamin D.

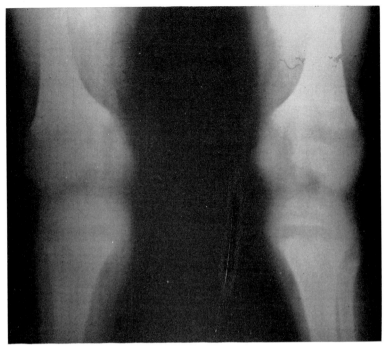

**Figure 12.1.** Rickets. This radiograph of both knee joints of a child, aged two years, shows widening and irregularity of the metaphyses. Following administration of vitamin D the growing ends of the long bones assumed a normal appearance. (*Courtesy of Dr. Lee A. Malmed*)

## OSTEOMALACIA

Osteomalacia is the adult counterpart of rickets. Since cartilage growth has ceased, the disease is characterized by a decreased concentration of hydroxyapatite in bone matrix.

CLINICAL FEATURES. The patient has vague aches and pains in the back, chest, pelvis and extremities. Spontaneous fractures or collapse of vertebrae may occur.

LABORATORY DIAGNOSIS. The serum calcium values are normal or at the lower limit of normal and the serum phosphorus concentrations are reduced from the normal adult levels of 3 to 4 mg. per 100 ml. Alkaline phosphatase activity is the same as in rickets.

TREATMENT is as in rickets.

## OSTEOPOROSIS

Osteoporosis is more common in women than in men and usually occurs after the fifth decade. The disease may occur in patients who have been immobilized for long periods in bed. It may also arise in younger women following removal of the ovaries. Because of this, it was thought that the withdrawal of estrogens was the cause of the osteoporosis but this has not been proved; only a small proportion of postmenopausal women develop osteoporosis. In many cases, no cause can be found.

HISTOPATHOLOGY. The trabeculae are reduced in size and number and the cortex is thin. The condition is often more advanced in the spine than elsewhere. The weakness of the bone leads to compression fractures of the vertebral bodies and fractures of other bones.

CLINICAL FEATURES. A frequent complaint is backache but sometimes a long bone or rib may fracture after minor trauma. The physical signs are loss of height and kyphosis.

TREATMENT. Immobilization should be avoided. Graded exercises should be given to all older patients confined to bed in order to prevent disuse atrophy. The diet should provide adequate proteins and vitamins and calcium gluconate or lactate may be given to supplement the dietary calcium intake. Estrogens are administered to female patients for three weeks out of four to prevent uterine bleeding. Male patients are given androgens.

## SCURVY

Scurvy is a disease which results from a deficiency of vitamin C in the diet. In infants, this occurs in a child aged from six months to one year who has been bottle-fed with boiled milk or milk substitutes since birth. In adults, the disease occurs in those whose diet is devoid of fresh fruits and vegetables.

The basic defect in scurvy is the failure of the various types of connective tissue cells to form their specific matrix. Fibroblasts are unable to form collagen; osteoblasts and odontoblasts do not synthesize osteoid and dentine respectively. Defects in the capillary wall occur in scurvy and result in hemorrhages.

CLINICAL FEATURES:

*Infantile scurvy.* The child holds his lower extremities flexed because they are swollen and exquisitely tender on movement. The costochondral junctions may be enlarged. The gingiva are swollen and bleeding occurs around erupted teeth; cutaneous hemorrhages are present.

*Adult scurvy.* There is bleeding from the gingiva only when the teeth are present. Cutaneous hemorrhages occur and there is pain and weakness of the lower extremities.

LABORATORY FINDINGS. When an adequate amount of vitamin C is being taken in the diet, it is excreted in the urine. If, after 200 mg. of vitamin C, none is excreted, this indicates that the body stores are depleted and that the patient is vitamin C deficient.

TREATMENT. Infants are given natural vitamin C as orange or tomato juice. Synthetic ascorbic acid up to 500 mg. daily is used in the treatment of adults.

## General Diseases of Bone

### OSTEOGENESIS IMPERFECTA

This disease is related to dentinogenesis imperfecta. The disease is usually present at birth although some cases do not arise until later in childhood.

HISTOPATHOLOGY. The essential feature is that osteoblastic activity is imperfect resulting in thin, delicate, bony trabeculae. The teeth show normal enamel and the dentine shows the presence of vascular canals.

CLINICAL FEATURES. The bones are extremely fragile and have a tendency to fracture. The fractures heal readily but the new bone is abnormal in structure. In this disease, the sclerae are blue. In addition to these characteristics, deafness and abnormal teeth which are identical in appearance with those of odontogenesis imperfecta also occur. The color of the teeth varies from yellowish-brown to bluish-black.

TREATMENT. No cure for the disease is known.

### CLEIDOCRANIAL DYSOSTOSIS

The etiology is unknown. The disease which is not always hereditary affects the ossification of the clavicles and membrane bones of the skull.

CLINICAL FEATURES. The clavicles may be entirely absent or only the central parts may be present. Because of this, the patient can make the shoulders touch in the midline. In the skull, there is often late closure of the fontanelles. The sutures also remain open and wormian bones are common. The maxillae, zygomatic bones and maxillary sinuses may be underdeveloped.

There is prolonged retention of deciduous teeth and some of the permanent dentition may erupt late or fail to erupt. Supernumerary teeth are common.

TREATMENT. No cure for the disease is known.

### OSTEOPETROSIS (ALBERS-SCHÖNBERG DISEASE)

Osteopetrosis is a disease of unknown etiology. It is often hereditary.

HISTOPATHOLOGY. Bone deposition occurs normally but there is a failure of bone resorption, resulting in sclerosis.

CLINICAL FEATURES. The disease usually manifests itself in the second decade of life. Because of the dense sclerosis of the bone, the individual bones tend to be brittle and fracture easily. The blood supply to the jaws is reduced as a result of the bone sclerosis and there is a marked tendency for osteomyelitis to occur following tooth extraction. Anemia is a common finding as a result of the replacement of myeloid tissue by bone.

LABORATORY FINDINGS. The serum phosphorus, calcium and alkaline phosphatase are normal.

RADIOGRAPHIC APPEARANCE. The bones show an increased density. The

11

medullary cavities are replaced by bone and the cortex is markedly thickened.

TREATMENT. No cure for the disease is known.

## ACHONDROPLASIA

In achondroplasia, the development of those bones which are preformed in cartilage is disturbed and this results in dwarfism. The condition, which is hereditary, is transmitted as a dominant characteristic.

HISTOPATHOLOGY. The cartilage columns in the long bones are irregular and fail to calcify properly. As a consequence, the patient's growth is retarded.

CLINICAL FEATURES. The achondroplastic dwarf has short arms and legs and a large head. The frontal bones are prominent, the maxillae retruded and the nasal bridge is depressed. The skull base which is preformed in cartilage is short. Dental anomalies and delayed eruption have been reported (Brook and Winter, 1970).

RADIOGRAPHIC APPEARANCE. The long bones are shorter than normal and the bones of the base of the skull fuse prematurely.

## INFANTILE CORTICAL HYPEROSTOSIS (CAFFEY'S DISEASE)

Caffey's disease is uncommon and tends to occur within the first three months of life. Although several causes have been suggested including a local vascular disorder and allergy, there is no agreement on its etiology.

CLINICAL FEATURES. The mandible, clavicles and ribs are the bones most commonly affected. Tender soft tissue swellings occur over the affected bone. When the mandible is involved, associated facial swelling occurs. The child may be febrile and hyperirritable. Radiographic examination shows the presence of cortical thickening.

The disease, for which there is no specific treatment, runs a benign course for weeks or months. Careful follow-up of some patients has shown a residual asymmetric deformity of the mandible.

## OSTEITIS DEFORMANS (PAGET'S DISEASE)

The disease is of unknown etiology. Possibly the bone disturbance may be due to an underlying vascular disorder since the bone in Paget's disease is highly vascular. Within the bone is an arterio-venous shunt which results in a low diastolic blood pressure; ultimately there is a tendency for the patient to die of cardiac failure.

HISTOPATHOLOGY. Both osteoclastic and osteoblastic phases occur in the disease. A characteristic feature of osteitis deformans is the presence of a mosaic pattern of the bone. This is caused by alternate resorption and deposition giving rise to reversal lines which stain with basophilic dyes.

CLINICAL FEATURES. The disease occurs in patients over the age of 40 and both sexes are affected. The skull progressively enlarges along with bowing of the legs and spinal curvature (Figure 12.2). The affected bones

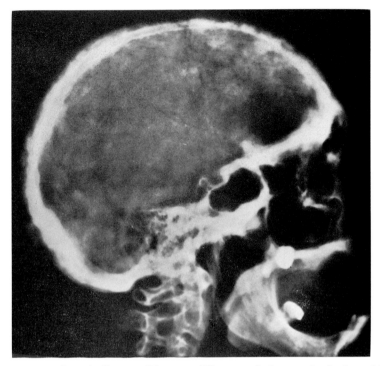

**Figure 12.2.** Paget's disease. There are diffuse osteolytic areas in the frontal bone and the typical "cotton-wool" appearance is present towards the posterior aspect of the skull. Male, aged 59 years.

are warm to touch and have a marked tendency to fracture. As a result of the deposition of bone around the internal auditory meatus and optic foramen, deafness and blindness may ensue. Some patients complain of bone pain or headaches. The disease affects the maxilla more commonly than the mandible and produces widening of the alveolus. Osteogenic sarcoma occurs in less than one percent of cases.

RADIOGRAPHIC APPEARANCE. At one stage in the disease, diffuse osteolytic areas occur in the skull resulting in osteoporosis circumscripta. The phase of osteoblastic activity is the most commonly recognized and gives rise to areas of bone sclerosis, the so-called "cotton-wool" appearance. The bones of the pelvis and the femurs are frequently affected. The teeth often show hypercementosis.

LABORATORY FINDINGS. The serum calcium and phosphorus are normal but the serum alkaline phosphatase is markedly raised.

TREATMENT. There is no specific therapy for osteitis deformans.

## FIBROUS DYSPLASIA OF BONE

This condition may be divided into two main types: the monostotic form where only one bone is involved, and the polyostotic form where many bones are involved.   In the latter, the lesions tend to have a unilateral distribution.   In some cases of polyostotic fibrous dysplasia occurring in young girls, pigmented patches on the skin and precocious puberty have been recorded (Albright's syndrome).   A familial form of fibrous dysplasia known as cherubism has been described.

HISTOPATHOLOGY.   The lesion is made up of fibroblasts and collagen in which areas of calcification or ossification occur.   Areas of liquefaction may occur in the connective tissue and give rise to cystic lesions.

CLINICAL FEATURES.   Fibrous dysplasia of bone occurs most commonly in young adults.   In the polyostotic form, there may be swelling and bowing of the long bones with spontaneous fracture.   Some cases are only discovered accidentally when radiographs are taken for some other purpose. Expansion and deformity of the jaws may occur when they are involved.

RADIOGRAPHIC APPEARANCE.   The medullary portions of the bone are rarefied and may present irregular trabeculations.   The cortical bone is usually thinned and often expanded.

LABORATORY FINDINGS.   The serum calcium and phosphorus are normal but the serum alkaline phosphatase may be raised.

TREATMENT.   Where there is marked deformity, the bone may be reduced in size by paring.

## LEONTIASIS OSSEA

In leontiasis ossea, there is hyperostosis of the facial bones.   It occurs in young adults and is thought to be a form of fibrous dysplasia which involves the facial bones.

## HYPERPARATHYROIDISM (p. 132)

# DISEASES OF JOINTS
## Classification of Arthritis

1. Polyarthritis of unknown etiology
   a. Rheumatoid arthritis
   b. Juvenile rheumatoid arthritis (Still's disease)
   c. Ankylosing spondylitis
2. Rheumatic fever
3. Degenerative joint disease (osteoarthritis, osteoarthrosis)
4. Associated with known biochemical abnormalities
   a. Gout
   b. Hemophilia

## POLYARTHRITIS OF UNKNOWN ETIOLOGY
### Rheumatoid Arthritis

Although this is a disease affecting primarily connective tissue, the joint inflammation is the dominant clinical manifestation.   The disease runs a chronic course leading to characteristic deformities and disability.

Women are affected three times as frequently as men. The most common age of onset is in the fourth decade but the disease may begin at any age, from early infancy to old age.

An autoimmune mechanism has been suggested in the pathogenesis of rheumatoid arthritis.

HISTOPATHOLOGY. Thickening of the articular soft tissues is characteristic of rheumatoid arthritis. Vascular granulation tissue also referred to as pannus forms in the synovial membrane and spreads over the cartilage which becomes eroded. In addition, the underlying bone may become eroded and osteoporotic. The pannus may be replaced by fibrous tissue leading to fibrous ankylosis of the joint.

The subcutaneous nodule is characteristic of rheumatoid arthritis. This consists of a central zone of fibrinoid material resulting from cellular necrosis. Surrounding this is a zone of primitive fibroblasts arranged in a palisade layer; this is in turn enveloped by a layer of fibrous tissue infiltrated with lymphocytes and plasma cells.

CLINICAL FEATURES. In adults, the small joints of the hands and feet become painful and swollen and the overlying skin is smooth, shiny and reddened. Malaise, weight loss and a feeling of fatigue and morning stiffness are common findings. Subcutaneous nodules are palpable about the elbow and the knee. Muscle weakness and atrophy are common.

If the disease is allowed to progress, permanent deformities appear. Subluxation of the metacarpophalangeal joint occurs and the hand is deviated towards the ulnar side.

Cardiac lesions, uveitis and secondary amyloidosis may also occur during the course of rheumatoid arthritis.

FELTY'S SYNDROME. This consists of rheumatoid arthritis, enlargement of the spleen (splenomegaly), leukopenia and usually anemia.

LABORATORY TESTS. The rheumatoid factor which is found in the serum of 70 to 80 percent of patients with rheumatoid arthritis is a macroglobulin with a molecular weight of about one million. It is demonstrated by a variety of serologic methods all depending on its affinity for $\gamma$ globulin.

Latex or bentonite particles coated with pooled human $\gamma$ globulin are agglutinated by rheumatoid factor. Sheep red cells coated with sub-hemolyzing amounts of rabbit antiserum against these cells will react with the patient's serum containing the rheumatoid factor.

The erythrocyte sedimentation rate is elevated during the active phases of the disease, and in addition, there is leukocytosis. Commonly the patient will have a moderately severe hypochromic anemia which is probably the result of an abnormality in the regulation of red cell production.

RADIOGRAPHIC EXAMINATION. Bone erosion, malalignment and subluxation are frequently observed on the radiographs of the small joints (Figure 12.3).

TREATMENT. Bed rest is important in severe cases. The affected joints should be rested by the use of plastic splints. Graded exercises are im-

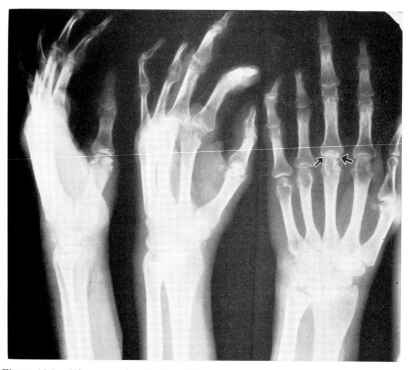

**Figure 12.3.** Rheumatoid arthritis. There is characteristic articular erosion with narrowing of the joint-space and demineralization best demonstrated at the metacarpophalangeal joint of the middle finger (arrows). Subluxations, such as seen at the distal interphalangeal joint of the fifth finger, are a common late feature. Note the amputated distal phalanx of the ring finger. (*Courtesy of Dr. Lee A. Malmed*)

portant to maintain muscle tone. Salicylates in the form of aspirin or sodium salicylate are the drugs most commonly employed. Gold salts have been used but toxicity reactions such as dermatitis and stomatitis are frequent.

### Juvenile Rheumatoid Arthritis (Still's Disease)

The disease may occur at any age up to 14 years. Girls are affected more than boys. Some children may have a prolonged fever before joint manifestations appear. Generalized lymphadenopathy, splenomegaly and a characteristic evanescent, salmon-colored morbilliform rash may be found. Destruction of ossification centers will interfere with growth. When the temporomandibular joint is involved, impaired mandibular growth occurs leading to a receding chin, a typical childhood deformity of rheumatoid arthritis.

LABORATORY TESTS. The rheumatoid factor is rarely found in the serum of children.

TREATMENT. This is similar to that in rheumatoid arthritis in adults.

## Ankylosing Spondylitis

About 90 percent of the patients with ankylosing spondylitis are males and the onset is usually in the late teens. The disease is progressive and affects the sacroiliac joints, the spinal apophyseal or synovial joints and the adjacent soft tissues. The cause is unknown.

HISTOPATHOLOGY. This resembles that of rheumatoid arthritis except that the disease results in bony ankylosis.

CLINICAL FEATURES. The earliest symptom is backache unrelieved by rest. As the disease progresses, back movement is restricted. In addition, the hip, shoulder and knee joints are involved. The temporomandibular joint is frequently affected and the jaw opening is restricted. An early finding is limitation of chest expansion to two or three cms. due to costo-vertebral joint involvement.

Iridocyclitis or iritis occurs in from one-third to one-fourth of patients and may lead to blindness.

LABORATORY TESTS. The erythrocyte sedimentation rate is frequently raised. In about one-third of the patients, mild hypochromic anemia is present.

RADIOGRAPHIC EXAMINATION. The earliest changes occur in the sacro-iliac joints with bone erosions developing at the margins; finally bony ankylosis occurs. In the spine, bony bridges (syndesmophytes) occur on the lateral and the anterior surfaces of the vertebrae. In advanced cases, the typical "bamboo spine" occurs (Figure 12.4).

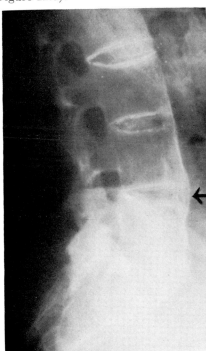

**Figure 12.4.** Ankylosing spondylitis. Lateral view of the lumbar spine demonstrating a "squaring-off" configuration of the vertebral bodies and calcification of the anterior longitudinal ligament (arrow) Male, aged 45 years. *(Courtesy of Dr. Lee A. Malmed)*

TREATMENT. Salicylates and phenylbutazone are given for relief of pain. Graduated exercises are of value. Splints are used for optimum positioning of joints threatened by ankylosis. In selected cases, surgery is employed for correction of deformities.

## RHEUMATIC FEVER (p. 48)

## DEGENERATIVE JOINT DISEASE (OSTEOARTHRITIS, OSTEOARTHROSIS)

Degenerative joint disease is more common in the elderly but may occur at an earlier age as a sequel to joint injury. The weight-bearing and intervertebral joints are the sites of predilection in both sexes. In postmenopausal women, the distal interphalangeal joints are frequently affected (Heberden's nodes).

PATHOLOGY. The articular cartilage degenerates and the subchondral bone becomes thickened and polished, this process being termed eburnation. Periosteal new bone formation occurs at the joint margins forming bony spurs or ridges called osteophytes.

CLINICAL FEATURES. A frequent complaint is joint pain particularly on weight-bearing or movement. In addition, the patient may experience stiffness after rest and aching when the weather is cold and damp. Physical examination may reveal limitation of movement of the joint with crepitation and spasm or atrophy of surrounding muscles. There are no systemic manifestations.

RADIOGRAPHIC EXAMINATION. In the early stages, the joint spaces narrow unevenly. Later, there is sclerosis of the bone ends with osteophyte formation.

TREATMENT. If the patient is overweight he should reduce. The affected joints should be rested as much as possible. Local heat and exercises to prevent muscle atrophy are important. Analgesics, particularly aspirin, are given to relieve pain. Surgical measures are of benefit when serious disability has resulted.

## ASSOCIATED WITH KNOWN BIOCHEMICAL ABNORMALITIES

### Gout

Gout is a metabolic disease characterized by an increased serum uric acid concentration. The latter probably results from excessive formation in the gouty individual. Females are rarely affected by the disease. In its early phases there are recurrent episodes of acute arthritis; in the late stages, tophi or deposits of urates occur in the tissues usually accompanied by the symptoms of chronic arthritis.

Increased uric acid formation occurs in leukemias and polycythemia giving rise to secondary gout.

HISTOPATHOLOGY. Urate crystals are frequently present in the joint structures. The tophus consists of urate crystals surrounded by a foreign body reaction.

CLINICAL FEATURES. In the early stages, the attacks are monarticular. The metatarsophalangeal joint of the big toe is commonly affected, the patient being awakened by severe pain. Movement of the toe is exquisitely painful and the patient cannot bear the weight of the bedclothes. Following the first attack, the patient is asymptomatic but later the attacks become more frequent and chronic gouty arthritis occurs. In chronic gout, tophi form over the cartilage of the ear and the olecranon.

TREATMENT. Colchicine is the drug of choice for acute gout. Between attacks, the patient should avoid high purine foods such as liver, kidneys and sardines. Uricosuric drugs such as probenecid, sulfinpyrazone and allopurinol decrease the serum uric acid concentration.

## Hemophilia (p. 102)

## SUGGESTED READING

*Primer on the Rheumatic Diseases*, 6th ed., Chicago, The Arthritis Foundation, 1964.

ACHONDROPLASIA

Brook, A. H., and Winter, G. B.: Dental anomalies in association with achondroplasia Brit. Dent. J., *129*, 519, 1970.

Chapter 13

# DISEASES OF THE NERVOUS SYSTEM

## THE CRANIAL NERVES

The cranial nerves may be affected by a number of pathologic processes:
1. Trauma, e.g. fracture of the base of the skull.
2. Vascular lesions, e.g. cerebral hemorrhage, thrombosis and embolism.
3. Inflammatory lesions, e.g. meningitis and encephalitis.
4. Neoplasms.

### The Olfactory Nerve (I)

Loss of the sense of smell (anosmia) may occur as a result of a fracture of the base of the skull or pressure by a tumor. The sense of smell is impaired with age.

### The Optic Nerve (II)

Light from the temporal side of the field of vision focuses on the nasal side of the retina and light from the nasal side of the field of vision focuses on the temporal side of the retina. In the optic chiasma, the fibers from the nasal sides of both retinae cross. A pituitary tumor in that region will press on these crossing fibers and result in impairment of vision in the temporal fields of vision (bitemporal hemianopsia).

Examination of the retina and optic disc is performed with the aid of the electric ophthalmoscope. Increased intracranial pressure due to a tumor will cause swelling of the optic disc (papilledema). Changes in the retina are produced in diseases such as hypertension, renal disease, blood dyscrasias and diabetes.

## The Oculomotor (III), Trochlear (IV) and Abducent (VI) Nerves

These nerves innervate the muscles which move the eyeball. The fourth nerve supplies the superior oblique muscle and the sixth nerve, the lateral rectus. All the other muscles are supplied by the third nerve which, in addition, sends fibers to the levator palpebrae superioris and controls the sphincter of the pupil and the ciliary muscle.

## CERVICAL SYMPATHETIC PARALYSIS (HORNER'S SYNDROME)

Damage to the cervical sympathetic as a result of an operation or a tumor will produce a small pupil (miosis), narrowed palpebral fissure (enophthalmos), drooping of the upper eyelid (ptosis) and lack of sweating on the affected side (anhydrosis).

## ARGYLL ROBERTSON PUPIL

This occurs in cerebrovascular syphilis and characteristically the pupil responds to accommodation but not to light.

## The Trigeminal Nerve (V)

The trigeminal nerve has both motor and sensory functions and subserves taste from the anterior $\frac{2}{3}$ of the tongue through the chorda tympani. The sensations of light touch, pressure and postural sense from the face are conducted to the principal sensory nucleus in the pons. Pain and temperature sensations from the face are conducted to the spinal cord. The motor nucleus of V lies in the pons.

## PARESTHESIA

Paresthesia is an abnormal sensation occurring in an area of the skin which the patient may variously describe as tingling, pins and needles, burning, coldness or a sense of water running over the skin. Paresthesia of an area of facial skin supplied by a branch of V may arise as the result of trauma or multiple sclerosis.

Pain arising from diseases of the eyes, teeth and paranasal sinuses is conveyed by branches of the trigeminal nerve. In addition, the trigeminal nerve is involved by a disorder of unknown etiology, paroxysmal trigeminal neuralgia or tic douloureux. The term "neuralgia" implies pain along the course of a nerve and is to be distinguished from neuritis which is inflammation of a nerve.

## PAROXYSMAL TRIGEMINAL NEURALGIA (TIC DOULOUREUX)
(see p. 169)

## The Facial Nerve (VII)

This nerve supplies the muscles of facial expression. Lacerations of the face may damage the branches of the facial nerve and result in paralysis of the muscles supplied by those branches. A malignant tumor of the parotid gland may also involve the facial nerve and cause facial paralysis. In addition, the seventh nerve may be affected by Bell's palsy.

## BELL'S PALSY

Bell's palsy is an acute lower motor neuron paralysis of the facial nerve which is of unknown etiology. It is believed to be the result of edema of the nerve in the facial canal.

CLINICAL FEATURES. The paralysis is usually preceded by pain in the ear or face. It involves all the facial muscles of one side of the face so that the patient cannot wrinkle the forehead, is unable to close the eye and when he attempts to do so, the eyeball rolls upwards. There is drooping of the corner of the mouth which results in drooling. Recovery usually occurs within six to eight weeks but may take up to one year. In some cases, permanent paralysis results. In an upper motor neuron lesion of VII when the injury lies between the motor cortex and the seventh nucleus, the patient can still wrinkle the forehead with the lower part of the face being paralyzed.

TREATMENT. Prednisolone and ACTH have been used. Physiotherapy is of value. When permanent deformity occurs, fascial slings are employed to support the sagging muscles. Nerve transplants have also been employed.

### The Auditory Nerve (VIII)

The eighth nerve is concerned with both hearing and vestibular function.

## DEAFNESS

There are two forms: conduction deafness and nerve deafness.

Conduction deafness is usually a sequel to inflammatory middle ear disease. It may occur with obstruction of the eustachian tube, otosclerosis or Paget's disease.

Nerve deafness may be congenital or may be caused by fractures of the temporal bone.

When tested with a tuning fork, it is found that in conduction deafness, bone conduction sounds louder than air conduction. In nerve deafness, acuity is reduced but air conduction is still the better.

## VESTIBULAR LESIONS

These will classically cause vertigo (dizziness) and unbalance.

## MENIERE'S DISEASE

This condition occurs more frequently in middle age and is more common in women than in men. It consists of deafness, tinnitus (ringing in the ears) and vertigo. It results from gross distention of the labyrinth by fluid.

TREATMENT is with antihistamines such as dimenhydrinate (Dramamine).

## The Glossopharyngeal Nerve (IX)

The nerve is motor to the stylopharyngeus muscle and secretomotor to the parotid gland. It supplies common sensation and taste to the posterior third of the tongue and the mucous membrane of the oropharynx.

## GLOSSOPHARYNGEAL NEURALGIA (see p. 170)

## The Vagus Nerve (X)

The tenth nerve has meningeal, auricular, pharyngeal and laryngeal branches and is the main parasympathetic supply to the thoracic and abdominal viscera.

## VAGAL PARALYSIS

If the patient is asked to say "Ah," normally the uvula moves backwards in the median plane, but in vagal paralysis it is deflected to the normal side. The nerve may be affected by diphtheritic paralysis which results in regurgitation of food through the nose and a nasal voice.

## The Accessory Nerve (XI)

The cranial root joins X and the fibers are distributed to the muscles of the pharynx, larynx and palate. The cervical root supplies the sterno-cleidomastoid and trapezius muscles. Injury to the nerve in the neck will result in paralysis of the sternocleidomastoid and trapezius muscles.

## The Hypoglossal Nerve (XII)

This nerve supplies the muscles of the tongue. Injury to the nerve during surgery will result in paralysis of that side of the tongue. When the tongue is protruded, it is noted to be wasted on the affected side and it also deviates to that side.

## HEADACHE

Although anatomically the head is the upper part of the body containing the mouth, sense organs and brain, the term "headache" is often restricted to pain felt within the cranial cavity and in the scalp. This is somewhat confusing to the student since the pain in one category of headache, Horton's headache (facial migrainous neuralgia), is felt in and around the eye.

### Categories of Headache

1. Vascular headache of the migraine type.
2. Muscle contraction headache (tension headache).
3. Recurrent daily headache following head injury.
4. Headache associated with arterial hypertension.
5. Vascular headache which accompanies fever, e.g. typhoid fever, influenza and malaria.

6. Headache referred from diseases of the nose, paranasal sinuses, eyes, ears and teeth.

7. Headache associated with intracranial disease, e.g. brain tumor, brain abscess, meningitis and hemorrhage.

Of the above categories, the first two are the most common and the last two are the least frequent.

The head pain of migraine, arterial hypertension and fever is the result of dilatation and distention of intracranial arteries.

## Migraine

This is a disorder of cerebral function which is commonly associated with visual disturbances, unilateral headache and vomiting. The cause of the disorder is cerebral vascular spasm later followed by dilatation of the affected vessels. Among the substances in the plasma which have been incriminated as possible causes of vascular headaches, are polypeptides and the kinins, particularly bradykinin. Another possible mechanism is that serotonin (5-hydroxytryptamine) activates some substance which affects the caliber of the blood vessels. Methysergide is used in the treatment of migraine by virtue of its action as a serotonin antagonist.

Individuals prone to migraine tend to be extremely conscientious. Premenstrual tension with fluid retention results in a tendency for migraine to be associated with this phase of the menstrual cycle.

CLINICAL FEATURES. The attack commences with unilateral headache experienced on waking in the morning, after a heavy sleep or at the weekend when tension is relieved. The headache becomes generalized and vomiting usually occurs as well as mild dizziness and photophobia. Paresthesia may occur in the face, arm and leg on the opposite side to the headache but around the mouth, the sensory disturbance is often bilateral. The attack terminates after a sleep and is followed by a diuresis.

TREATMENT. When attacks are frequent, phenobarbital and chlordiazepoxide (Librium) are prescribed. Ergotamine by injection will often abort an attack. It is, however, contraindicated in hypertensive, arteriosclerotic and pregnant patients.

## Muscle Contraction Headaches

These headaches occur in tense individuals and are the result of muscle spasm. The pain which may be unilateral or bilateral in character is felt in the temporal, occipital, parietal and frontal regions. On palpation, painful nodules may be felt in the muscles.

TREATMENT. Manipulation and stretching of the nuchal muscles is of value. The patient is reassured. Aspirin and phenobarbital are prescribed.

## Head Injury

Following a head injury, a generalized headache will result and slowly subside. The importance of gradual, steady increase in activity is now well-recognized in the prevention of prolonged headache after a head injury (p. 185).

## Arterial Hypertension

Severe hypertension will produce a severe headache which occurs in the early morning. Papilledema (choked disc) is often present in such patients together with a diastolic pressure of 140 mms. or more. It is important to give hypotensive treatment.

## Fever

This type of headache will subside on treatment of the fever.

## Referred Pain

Diseases of the nose, paranasal sinuses, eyes, ears and teeth may cause headache.

## Intracranial Disease

The headache associated with a brain tumor is a steady, dull, aching pain situated deeply which tends to be more intense in the morning. Coughing or straining at stool may aggravate the headache. The headache is rarely as intense as that associated with migraine, ruptured cerebral aneurysm or meningitis. It is uncommon for it to interfere with sleep.

## FACIAL PAIN

Stimuli of sufficient intensity when applied to a pain receptor are perceived as pain by the brain. Pain receptors are free nerve endings, most of non-medullated fibers. These sensory nerve endings occur as two types: large diameter fibers for the rapid conduction of sharp pain, and small diameter fibers for the slower conduction of dull pain.

## Causes of Facial Pain

1. *Temporomandibular Joint Dysfunction*
2. *Dental Disease*
   a. Pulpal
   b. Periodontal
   c. Gingival
3. *Diseases of the Ear, Nose and Throat*
   a. Acute sinusitis
   b. Otitis media
   c. Neoplasms of the sinuses
   d. Carcinoma of the nasopharynx
4. *Diseases of the Eye*
   a. Corneal ulceration
   b. Iritis
   c. Glaucoma

5. *Cervical Disc Lesions*
6. *Cardiac Disease*
   a. Coronary ischemia
   b. Coronary occlusion (infarction)
7. *Neuralgia*
   a. Primary (no obvious gross pathology)
      Paroxysmal trigeminal neuralgia (tic douloureux)
      Glossopharyngeal neuralgia
      Facial (periodic) migrainous neuralgia
      Atypical facial neuralgia
      Postherpetic neuralgia
   b. Secondary or symptomatic (nerve involved by growth, scar, injury or infection)

## Temporomandibular Joint Dysfunction

Although the temporomandibular joint may be affected by such conditions as osteoarthritis, rheumatoid arthritis, fractures, ankylosis and rarely by neoplasms, the most common temporomandibular joint disorder is a pain-dysfunction syndrome. In the past, discrepancies in occlusion or maxillomandibular relationships, or both, have been considered to be the etiologic factors of the pain-dysfunction syndrome. It has recently been suggested that the most common cause of this syndrome is muscle fatigue produced by chronic oral habits such as clenching or grinding of the teeth associated with underlying nervous tension (Laskin, 1969). Organic changes such as occlusal disharmonies, degenerative arthritis and degenerative changes in the muscles of mastication that accompany the long-term spasm may result and tend to make the condition self-perpetuating.

CLINICAL FEATURES. Pain is of unilateral origin, the muscles of mastication are tender, the temporomandibular joint makes a clicking or popping noise, and jaw function is limited. The diagnosis is confirmed by the absence of clinical, radiographic or biochemical evidence of organic changes in the temporomandibular joint and a lack of tenderness when the joint is palpated via the external auditory meatus.

TREATMENT. Occlusal grinding, the insertion of a removable appliance and bite rehabilitation are employed. Analgesics are given for the relief of pain and tranquilizers are prescribed to relieve the underlying tension.

## Dental Disease

This is one of the most common causes of facial pain. Its diagnosis and treatment are dealt with in the dental textbooks. It should, however, be remembered that pain of pulpal and periodontal origin characteristically does not cross the midline and that gingivitis is the only dental condition which causes pain all around the mouth.

## Diseases of the Ear, Nose and Throat

### ACUTE SINUSITIS

In maxillary sinusitis, a dull, aching pain is felt in the cheek and the maxillary teeth and may also be referred above the eye. In ethmoidal sinusitis, the pain is medial and deep to the eye. In frontal sinusitis, the pain is in the forehead, above the eyebrow. In infection of the sphenoid sinus, the pain is deep behind the eye, in the occiput and sometimes is referred to the vertex of the skull. In acute frontal and maxillary sinusitis, pain is typically not present in the early morning. It usually appears one to two hours after rising, increases for three or four hours and becomes less severe in the late afternoon and evening.

Chronic sinusitis gives rise to a chronic nasal discharge and not facial pain.

TREATMENT. An attempt is made to reduce the inflammation of the mucous membrane of the sinus by means of steam inhalations and nasal drops containing a vasoconstrictor. Antibiotics may be administered but this is usually unnecessary.

### OTITIS MEDIA

Infection of the middle ear results in severe pain which is felt in the ear.

TREATMENT. Antibiotics are administered. Myringotomy (incision of the drum) may be necessary to allow the pus to drain.

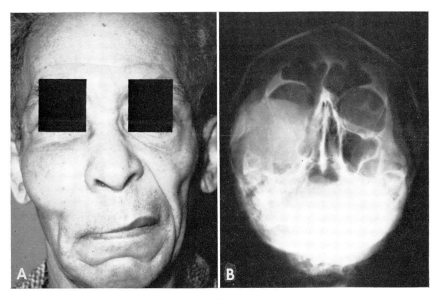

**Figure 13.1A.** Carcinoma of the antrum. The patient, a male aged 54 years, was complaining of swelling of the right cheek associated with pain and a bloody discharge from the right nostril. **B.** The radiograph shows a mass in the right antrum which has destroyed the antral wall and orbital floor.

12

## NEOPLASMS OF THE SINUSES

Malignant disease of the paranasal sinuses may give rise to pain, anesthesia or a bloody nasal discharge (Figure 13.1).

TREATMENT. Both surgery and radiotherapy are employed.

## CARCINOMA OF THE NASOPHARYNX

A carcinoma of the nasopharynx may give rise to Trotter's syndrome. This consists of neuralgic pain in the lower jaw, side of the head, tongue and ear associated with middle ear deafness and defective mobility of the soft palate on the same side. More common symptoms of a carcinoma of the nasopharynx are malignant involvement of the upper deep cervical lymph nodes, nasal obstruction, epistaxis and headache.

TREATMENT. Both surgery and radiotherapy are employed.

### Diseases of the Eye

The pain which occurs in diseases of the eye is felt mainly in the area supplied by the ophthalmic division of the trigeminal nerve.

## CORNEAL ULCERATION

This may result from trauma or infection. The conjunctival vessels are injected and pain, photophobia, lacrimation and blepharospasm (spasm of the eyelids) are present.

TREATMENT consists of the instillation of antibiotic eyedrops. Atropine drops may be instilled to dilate the pupil and rest the iris and ciliary body.

## IRITIS

The iris may become inflamed from infections of the cornea, from systemic disorders such as gonorrhea, syphilis, tuberculosis and Behçet's syndrome and from unknown causes (idiopathic). The iris forms part of the uveal tract which nourishes the eyeball and consists of the iris, ciliary body and choroid. Because of their close association, inflammation of one part frequently results in inflammation of the other two.

CLINICAL FEATURES. The patient complains of pain, photophobia, lacrimation and interference with vision. The vessels around the cornea which are normally not visible become distended and appear diffuse and purplish red. The iris markings become indistinct and its color changes because of congestion and edema. Because of the changes in the iris, the pupil is contracted and reacts sluggishly to light.

TREATMENT. Atropine is used to dilate the pupil and put the iris and ciliary body at rest. General infections are also treated when present as these may be the causative factors.

## GLAUCOMA

In glaucoma, intraocular pressure increases and, if untreated, will cause atrophy of the retinal ganglion cells and produce visual impairment.

CLINICAL FEATURES. The patient in the early stages of the condition complains of haloes around lights. This is followed by rapid failure of sight and severe pain in the eye sometimes accompanied by headache which may be associated with nausea and vomiting. The lids are swollen and edematous. The bulbar conjunctiva is congested and edematous. The cornea is cloudy and there is intense circumcorneal injection of a dark red color. The pupil is dilated, oval and immobile. Pressure with the fingers over the closed lids will confirm the increase in intraocular tension.

TREATMENT. An attempt is made to reduce intraocular pressure by means of instillation of pilocarpine eyedrops. An iridectomy is often indicated to prevent recurrence of the condition.

### Cervical Disc Lesions

The skin over the angle of the mandible is supplied by C 2 and 3 and pain in this region may occasionally be the result of pressure on a nerve root by a prolapsed intervertebral disc. The patient will have pain on movement of the neck and spasm of the associated muscles.

TREATMENT. This consists of rest in bed and analgesics followed by the wearing of a plastic collar if the pain does not subside.

### Cardiac Disease

#### CORONARY ISCHEMIA

Rarely patients may complain of pain in the jaws following exercise; this is caused by coronary ischemia.

#### CORONARY OCCLUSION

This can, on occasion, give rise to pain referred to the jaws.

### Neuralgia

Neuralgia is pain along the course of a nerve and may conveniently be divided into primary types where there is no obvious pathology and secondary or symptomatic types where a pathologic lesion can be demonstrated.

#### PRIMARY NEURALGIA

#### Paroxysmal Trigeminal Neuralgia

Although this form of neuralgia may occur as a symptom of cerebral tumor, an aneurysm, Paget's disease of the skull, a cholesteatoma or multiple sclerosis, the majority of cases are idiopathic. There are many theories concerning its causation, the current one being that the trigeminal nerve is stretched as it passes over the apex of the petrous bone which is higher on the affected side (Gardner and Dohn, 1966). It is postulated that the longstanding pressure produces an artificial synapse with a short circuiting effect. In addition, proliferative changes in the myelin sheaths of affected ganglia on electron microscopy have been described (Beaver et al., 1965).

CLINICAL FEATURES. Women are affected twice as often as men and the right side of the face is more commonly affected than the left. The second and third divisions of the trigeminal nerve are commonly affected but not the first. The condition may be encountered from the age of 30 but the commonest age of onset is between 60 and 70. The pain, which is characteristically severe and paroxysmal, may be described as stabbing, electrical, burning, explosive, searing and cutting. Paroxysms of pain last only for a few seconds but the actual bout may last for several hours with varying intervals of freedom from pain between actual paroxysms. Between paroxysms, the patient may be symptom-free or may have soreness or a dull ache in the affected area. The bouts themselves may continue for days or weeks. The patient will often state that touching or shaving a particular area will precipitate an attack and this is referred to as a "trigger zone." However, trigger zones are not diagnostic of the condition. Often the zone, when tested, is in a refractory state and, hence, a negative result does not exclude a diagnosis of paroxysmal trigeminal neuralgia.

TREATMENT. Drugs such as carbamezapine (Tegretol) or phenytoin sodium may be prescribed. Alcohol injection of peripheral nerves and the Gasserian ganglion have been used and will give relief for up to 18 months but may have to be repeated. In addition, peripheral neurectomies, cutting the entire preganglionic sensory root and medullary tractotomy are employed by neurosurgeons.

### Glossopharyngeal Neuralgia

The pain of glossopharyngeal neuralgia is similar in character to paroxysmal trigeminal neuralgia. It originates in the tonsillar fossa and may be referred to the ear. Spasms of pain may be initiated by swallowing.

TREATMENT. Dilantin or Tegretol may be tried but if this is unsuccessful, division of the nerve near the medulla is employed.

### Facial (Periodic) Migrainous Neuralgia

This form of neuralgia has also been termed "sphenopalatine neuralgia," "histamine cephalalgia," "cluster headache" and "alarm clock headache." It is more common in males than females and in the majority of patients, the symptoms first appear between the ages of 20 and 40 years.

CLINICAL FEATURES. The pain is of sudden onset and is extremely severe. During an attack, which may last from one half to two hours, the pain is experienced in and around the eye. The paroxysms are often nocturnal and characteristically will awaken the patient from his sleep at the same time in the early hours of the morning. There may be redness of the corresponding eye with increased lacrimation and the nostril on the same side may feel blocked. The patient may have the pain every night for several weeks, then a period of remission which may last from several months to many years.

TREATMENT. Ergotamine by mouth or injection is the treatment of choice and must be given regularly two or three times a day. It is given for five or six days, stopping on the sixth or seventh day of each week to determine whether a spontaneous remission has occurred. In hypertensive, arteriosclerotic and pregnant patients ergotamine is contraindicated and aspirin or codeine by the oral route should be tried.

### Atypical Facial Neuralgia

This is thought to be psychogenic in origin and is frequently associated with depression.

CLINICAL FEATURES. This condition occurs usually in young or middle-aged women and gives a dull aching pain, often in the maxillary region which may cross the midline. The pain is continuous but often becomes more severe towards evening. It does not interfere with eating or sleeping and may last for months or years.

TREATMENT. The pain can often be relieved with antidepressant and tranquilizer drugs. When the associated symptoms suggest severe endogenous depression, electroconvulsive therapy is sometimes needed, particularly if the pain and depression resist drug treatment. There remains, however, a small proportion of cases in which, despite treatment, the pain continues unabated and no organic cause is ever discovered.

### Postherpetic Neuralgia

In some patients, a severe neuralgia may follow an attack of herpes zoster. The herpes zoster virus which is identical with that causing chickenpox (varicella) may involve a posterior root ganglion, the gasserian ganglion or the geniculate ganglion. In many patients with herpes zoster, there is no apparent predisposing cause but in some patients, Hodgkin's disease and leukemia may be associated with this condition.

CLINICAL FEATURES. There is usually pain in the affected root or roots followed a few days later by erythema and a vesicular eruption in the approximate area of skin. The vesicles dry up and form crusts which drop off leaving pitted scars.

Two forms of herpes zoster seen in the region of the head are:

*Ophthalmic (Gasserian) Herpes.* Herpes zoster may affect the ophthalmic division of the fifth nerve and lead to corneal ulceration and scarring over the forehead. Some patients may have postherpetic neuralgia following ophthalmic herpes.

TREATMENT. An antibiotic cream can be applied to the skin lesions to prevent secondary infection but this is often unnecessary. Antibiotic drops may be instilled into the affected eye. Analgesics are given for the pain. If postherpetic neuralgia should occur, the pain is often very severe and analgesics may not relieve it. The treatment of this form of neuralgia is unsatisfactory.

*Geniculate Herpes (Ramsay Hunt Syndrome)*. This presents with pain in the ear followed by a vesicular eruption in the external auditory meatus and facial paralysis of the lower motor neuron type. Geniculate neuralgia may follow geniculate herpes and results in severe pain in the ear.

TREATMENT. Geniculate neuralgia may be treated by cutting the nervus intermedius in the internal auditory meatus.

## SECONDARY NEURALGIA

In secondary types of neuralgia, the nerve is involved by a new growth, a scar, an injury or infection and pain is felt in the distribution of the affected nerve. Paresthesia and anesthesia may accompany or follow the pain.

# INFECTIONS OF THE NERVOUS SYSTEM
## Meningitis

This is an acute inflammation of the meninges of the brain or spinal cord or both. It can be caused by bacteria, viruses or fungi. Only the bacterial and viral forms will be considered. Bacterial meningitis, except that caused by tubercle bacilli, generally is characterized by a purulent exudate.

### Cerebrospinal Fluid

The cerebrospinal fluid (CSF) is secreted by the choroid plexuses in the lateral, third and fourth ventricles; it circulates through the ventricular system of the brain and the subarachnoid space before being reabsorbed into the dural venous system. In the normal patient, the CSF has the following characteristics: clear and colorless in appearance; pressure, 70–200 mms. $H_2O$; cells/cu. mm. 0–5; protein, 15–45 mg./100 ml.; glucose, 50–75 mg./100 ml.

CSF can be withdrawn by lumbar puncture and its various constituents analyzed; in addition, culture of the fluid will reveal the causative organism of the meningitis. In purulent meningitis, the CSF is purulent and contains several thousand polymorphs, increased protein and greatly decreased glucose. The CSF in tuberculous meningitis is clear or opalescent, contains predominantly lymphocytes and the protein is raised.

### PURULENT MENINGITIS

*Neisseria meningitidis* (meningococcus), pneumococcus and *Haemophilus influenzae* are the most common causative organisms. Purulent meningitis results either from primary infection of the meninges and CSF or, less commonly, by the extension of infection from the middle ear or frontal sinuses or from a cerebral abscess.

CLINICAL FEATURES. The onset, which is usually acute, is characterized by fever, headache and vomiting accompanied by a stiff neck. In children, convulsions may occur. The patient may lapse into coma. There is pain on attempting to flex the neck and on attempting to extend the knee joint when the thigh has been flexed as far as possible on the abdomen (Kernig's sign).

TREATMENT is the appropriate antibiotic.

## TUBERCULOUS MENINGITIS

It occurs most commonly in children and young adults and is always secondary to tuberculosis elsewhere in the body. In the child, the initial symptoms are irritability, drowsiness, anorexia, constipation, vomiting and slight fever. As the disease progresses, fever increases and stupor and convulsions occur. In older patients, changes in behavior and complaints of headache are prominent.

Examination of the CSF is necessary for diagnosis, as are chest x-ray and tuberculin test. In some cases, tubercles can be seen with an ophthalmoscope on the choroid of the eye.

TREATMENT is with antituberculous drugs.

## VIRAL MENINGITIS

The symptoms of viral meningitis are the same as those for purulent meningitis. The diagnosis depends on the examination of the CSF; usually 100–1000 lymphocytes/cu.mm. are present.

### Virus Infections

Many viruses are capable of affecting the nervous system but some of the commonest ones are poliomyelitis (see following), herpes zoster (p. 6), lymphocytic choriomeningitis, herpes simplex, mumps (p. 8), Coxsackie and ECHO viruses.

There is no specific treatment for virus infections but the prognosis is usually good.

### Poliomyelitis

The causative agent is a small, RNA virus which belongs to the enterovirus family, a subgroup of the picornaviruses. Polioviruses exist in three immunologic types, type I most commonly being associated with epidemics. The virus enters the body by way of the oropharynx. Within three to four days following exposure, the virus is present in the throat, blood and feces. Invasion of the nervous system is thought to be by way of the bloodstream. The characteristic lesions of poliomyelitis are found in the gray matter and particularly the anterior horn cells of the spinal cord and the motor nuclei of the brain stem.

CLINICAL FEATURES. There are two main types, the minor illness and the major illness. Patients with the minor illness usually have slight fever, malaise, headache, sore throat and vomiting. These symptoms may last two to three days and may then disappear or the major illness may develop. In the latter, there are increased headache, stiff neck, back and muscle pains. In paralytic cases, weakness of various muscles and loss of superficial and deep reflexes occur. The legs tend to be involved more than the arms. In about fifteen percent of patients there is involvement of the cranial nuclei and muscles of the face, pharynx, larynx and tongue may be paralyzed. Respiratory paralysis occurs in some patients. Examination of the CSF will show increased cells, polymorphs in the early stages and later, lymphocytes. In addition, the protein content may be increased.

PROPHYLAXIS. Poliomyelitis is now a preventable disease and immunization is recommended for children and young adults. There are two methods of administration, the live attenuated virus (Sabin) given orally and the formalin-inactivated virus (Salk) injected parenterally.

TREATMENT. In the preparalytic stage, rest is essential as it has been shown that strenuous exercise increases the likelihood of paralysis. Analgesics are given to control pain. If paralysis does occur, relief of muscle pain and spasm is best accomplished by the frequent application of hot, moist packs. If respiratory paralysis occurs, the patient may have to be placed in a tank respirator. A tracheostomy may be necessary to assist breathing and to clean out secretions from the bronchial tract.

### Neurosyphilis

Syphilis may involve the brain, meninges or spinal cord. Some patients are asymptomatic, a positive S.T.S. (serologic test for syphilis) being found on routine examination. Examination of the CSF will enable the diagnosis of neurosyphilis to be made. The symptomatic forms of neurosyphilis are meningovascular syphilis, general paresis and tabes dorsalis. The S.T.S. is usually reactive in these forms.

## MENINGOVASCULAR SYPHILIS

This form which involves the meninges or the cerebral blood vessels may occur in localized or generalized forms. Cranial nerve palsies may develop in mild cases. In more severe cases, hemiplegia may occur.

## GENERAL PARESIS

In this form, the inflammatory process involves the cerebral cortex and overlying meninges. The early symptoms are headaches and memory defects. As the disease progresses, personality changes occur and the patient becomes slovenly in his habits.

## TABES DORSALIS

There is progressive degeneration of the ascending sensory neurons in the posterior columns of the spinal cord together with the posterior sensory ganglia and nerve roots.

CLINICAL FEATURES. "Lightning pains" are common and characteristic. They are stabbing in character, last a few seconds and occur in the lower limbs. The patient notices that he is unsteady in the dark when he can no longer rely on his sight for orientation. He tends to walk with a wide base because of his unsteadiness. The patient may complain of incontinence. Ulcers which fail to heal may occur on the feet.

Examination usually reveals diminution or absence of ankle and knee reflexes and, in addition, the Argyll Robertson pupil occurs frequently. The latter is a small irregular pupil which reacts to accommodation but not to light.

TREATMENT of neurosyphilis is with penicillin or erythromycin if the patient is allergic to penicillin.

## SYRINGOMYELIA

This is a condition of unknown etiology in which there is cystic degeneration of the gray matter of the spinal cord around the central canal. The pain and temperature fibers which cross the spinal cord in that area are interrupted as is the reflex arc. The result is dissociated sensory loss with loss of pain and temperature sensation and preservation of touch, and vibration and position loss. There is, in addition, loss of reflexes and wasting of the small muscles of the hand. The patient may complain of pain in the arms and weakness of the legs.

TREATMENT. Radiotherapy to the affected part of the cord has been employed.

## MYASTHENIA GRAVIS

Patients with myasthenia gravis have abnormal fatigue of striated muscle and rapid recovery after rest. The disease is caused by a defect in acetylcholine metabolism. Recent evidence suggests that myasthenia gravis is an autoimmune disease. Under the age of 30 years, women are more affected than men but after that age, there is male preponderance.

CLINICAL FEATURES. The most common early manifestations are ptosis (drooping of the upper eyelid) and diplopia (double vision). At first, the weakness is transient but worse toward the end of the day or after exercise of the affected muscles. Spontaneous exacerbations and remissions occur. Some patients may have difficulties in speech, chewing and swallowing and respiratory paralysis may occur.

TREATMENT is with the anticholinesterase drugs such as neostigmine (Prostigmin) and pyridostigmine (Mestinon).

## EPILEPSY

Epilepsy is a disorder of the nervous system which is characterized by the spontaneous abnormal discharge of nerve cells. For convenience, epilepsy may be divided into two categories:

1. *Idiopathic*—no apparent cause; most cases occur before the age of 20 years.
2. *Symptomatic*—associated with disease, e.g. tumor or scar following a head injury.

A further classification of epilepsy which is employed is:
1. *General*
   a. Grand mal
   b. Petit mal
2. *Focal*
   a. Psychomotor epilepsy
   b. Jacksonian and focal motor epilepsy

### Grand Mal (Major) Epilepsy

Grand mal epilepsy is characterized by attacks of loss of consciousness associated with convulsive movements. The sequence of events includes:

1. An aura which may be motor, sensory or psychic.
2. Tonic stage at the onset of which consciousness is lost. The patient falls to the ground with all the muscles in a state of rigid spasm. The tonic stage lasts approximately one minute and during this stage the breathing is held in abeyance resulting in cyanosis.
3. Clonic stage during which there are convulsive movements of muscles. The jaw and tongue may be involved so that the saliva becomes foamy and the tongue may be bitten. Involuntary micturition occurs.
4. Coma which may last from minutes to several hours. At this stage, the corneal and tendon reflexes are absent and extensor plantar responses are present.
5. On recovery, there is severe headache.

## STATUS EPILEPTICUS

Status epilepticus is the term employed for a continuing series of grand mal attacks occurring over hours or days in which the patient remains unconscious between attacks, the temperature gradually rises as high as 105° F and a fatal outcome may result.

### Petit Mal

Petit mal attacks are characterized by a loss of consciousness without convulsions, except for minor movements such as blinking. During childhood, petit mal attacks occur as brief interruptions of consciousness in which the patient stops what he is doing or saying for a few seconds and then carries on, or he may fall to the ground. These attacks are associated with bilaterally synchronous three-per-second spike and wave activity in the electroencephalogram which can be precipitated by hyperventilation.

### Psychomotor Epilepsy

Psychomotor epilepsy is characterized by dreamy states and periods of automatism. During an attack, the patient may carry out some purposive movements such as undressing or searching the floor and has no recollection of the attack after it has passed.

## Jacksonian and Focal Motor Epilepsy

The Jacksonian attack begins with localized jerky twitching on one side, such as the thumb. The jerky movements may then spread up the forearm and into the arm of the same side. In adults, Jacksonian epilepsy is frequently caused by a cerebral tumor. Other focal motor seizures involve gross movements of the arms or legs without the typical Jacksonian spread.

TREATMENT OF EPILEPSY. Phenobarbital and dilantin (diphenylhydantoin sodium) are used in the treatment of grand mal. Dilantin causes hyperplasia of the gingiva and in some patients, nystagmus and hirsutism. Zarontin (ethosuximide) is the drug of choice for petit mal seizures. Status epilepticus can be terminated by intravenous sodium amytal. Tongue biting is prevented by using a padded wooden tongue depressor.

DENTAL MANAGEMENT OF EPILEPTICS. Epileptics can be adequately treated using local anesthesia. Some authorities prefer to administer a general anesthetic for oral surgery in order to prevent a seizure during treatment.

## INTRACRANIAL HEMORRHAGE

Intracranial hemorrhage may be:
1. Extradural  ⎫
2. Subdural   ⎬ traumatic in origin
3. Subarachnoid
4. Intracerebral

### Extradural Hemorrhage

This condition arises as a result of a temporal or parietal fracture with laceration of the middle meningeal artery and vein.

CLINICAL FEATURES. The patient has a history of a head injury with loss of consciousness followed by a fairly rapid recovery. After a "lucid interval" there is gradually increasing coma with progressive hemiplegia and a fixed pupil on the side of the hematoma. Death ensues if the clot is not removed.

TREATMENT. This consists of ligation of the bleeding vessel.

### Subdural Hemorrhage

Subdural hemorrhage occurs mostly in elderly patients and may follow a trivial injury. The blood comes from veins and oozes into the subdural space where it clots.

CLINICAL FEATURES. After a period of weeks following the injury, the patient complains of headaches and giddiness. These symptoms are associated with slowness of thinking, confusion and alteration in the personality.

TREATMENT. This consists of evacuation of the clot.

## Subarachnoid Hemorrhage

Cerebral aneurysms which are usually congenital but sometimes develop as the result of atheroma, tend to occur in and around the circle of Willis. They provide by far the commonest source of subarachnoid hemorrhage.

CLINICAL FEATURES. The patient experiences a sudden severe headache preceding loss of consciousness with the rapid development of stiffness of the neck.

TREATMENT. Absolute bed rest is prescribed together with sedation. If the patient survives the original episode, surgical treatment is carried out to prevent recurrence of the hemorrhage.

## Intracerebral Hemorrhage

This constitutes one form of stroke or cerebrovascular accident; the other causes are cerebral thrombosis and embolism.

# CEREBROVASCULAR ACCIDENTS

Cerebrovascular accidents are usually the result of atheroma or arterial hypertension. The blood supply of the brain is from the carotid and vertebral-basilar system of arteries. The latter is responsible for supplying the brain stem. A lesion of the carotid system produces unilateral neurologic signs affecting the opposite side of the body; a lesion of the vertebral-basilar system frequently produces bilateral signs. Most cerebrovascular accidents involve the middle cerebral artery or one of its branches. The interruption of the blood supply to part of the brain will produce softening of the affected area followed by neurologic dysfunction.

## Cerebral Atherosclerosis

Atherosclerosis of the cerebral vessels is most frequently found in patients over the age of sixty years. Arterial thrombosis is one of the most common causes of cerebrovascular accidents and this usually follows atherosclerosis of the affected vessel. However, slowing of the circulation (as in episodes of systemic hypotension) and increased viscosity of the blood (as in polycythemia) serve as contributory causes.

## Hypertensive Cerebral Hemorrhage

It is believed that the factors involved in hypertensive cerebral hemorrhage are a primary degeneration of the walls of the affected vessels and, following that, a sudden increase in pressure of the diseased vessel with tearing of the vessel wall. The bleeding in spontaneous intracerebral hemorrhage usually occurs deep in the cerebral hemispheres.

Occasionally, the hemorrhage may rupture into the ventricular system and thus accounts for the presence of blood in the cerebrospinal fluid. Cerebral hemorrhage is frequently fatal.

## Cerebral Embolism

The usual sources of emboli in cerebral embolism are from fibrillating atria, myocardial infarcts and the vegetations of subacute bacterial endocarditis.

CLINICAL FEATURES. Cerebrovascular accidents are of all degrees of severity. The worst forms cause immediate loss of consciousness but the important feature is that the affected limbs fall more heavily to the bed than those on the unaffected side. There is puffing of one side of the mouth or conjugate deviation of the eyes so that the patient "looks at his lesion." The classical signs of upper motor neuron lesion develop only after an interval of some hours or days. In addition, a stroke may give rise to numbness, blindness, diplopia, dizziness and speech disturbances (aphasia). The latter is a frequent accompaniment if the left side of the brain is affected. The least severe strokes present as only the slightest weakness of a limb, with mild headaches and a little confusion.

TREATMENT. When the patient is in coma, maintenance of the airway is important often with the administration of oxygen. Intravenous fluids are given followed by nasogastric fluids. An indwelling catheter is passed into the bladder to prevent distention of that organ. Passive movements of the limbs are carried out together with massage to prevent contractures. The patient is later encouraged to move his limbs voluntarily. Most hemiplegics can learn to walk again.

## Dental Management of the Post-CVA Patient

If there is any doubt about the patient's physical status, a medical consultation is desirable. No elective dental treatment is given for at least six months after the episode. Appointments are kept as short as possible. Sedation with a hypnotic is useful but should be used with great care as heavy sedation depresses the cerebral circulation and can initiate cerebral thrombosis.

## DEMYELINATING DISEASES

### Multiple Sclerosis

This disease is characterized by plaques of myelin destruction in the white matter of the spinal cord and brain. The etiology of multiple sclerosis is still unknown although autoimmune disease, copper deficiency and infection by a virus have all been implicated. The disease is more common in temperate climates. Most patients manifest symptoms between 20 and 40 years of age.

CLINICAL FEATURES. The chronic form of the disease is the most common variety. The patient may complain of weakness or loss of control of the limbs. There may be numbness or tingling in the hands or feet which may also be painful. The patient may experience increased frequency or urgency of micturition.

A common initial symptom is sudden loss of vision in one eye (retrobulbar neuritis) or double-vision (diplopia) and these symptoms frequently remit.

In some patients, there is slow progression of the disease resulting in paralysis of the legs, ataxia of the arms due to tremor or postural loss and urinary infection. In the well-established disease, the tendon reflexes are exaggerated and an extensor Babinski response (an upgoing great toe) is present; the abdominal reflexes are absent.

TREATMENT. There is no specific treatment but corticotrophin is claimed to be helpful in acute relapses.

## EXTRAPYRAMIDAL DISORDERS

The extrapyramidal system is comprised of the extrapyramidal motor neurons and the basal ganglia. Diseases of the latter cause disorders of muscle tone and movements. There is muscle rigidity and involuntary movements occur.

### Paralysis Agitans (Parkinson's Disease)

Paralysis agitans usually occurs between the ages of 40 and 65; it is the result of degeneration occurring mainly in the substantia nigra. Postencephalitic parkinsonism and arteriosclerotic parkinsonism have a similar clinical picture to paralysis agitans but their etiologies are different.

CLINICAL FEATURES. The patient has a rigid facial expression with slowness of movement and a stooped posture. The gait is shuffling and the arms are held to the side. There is rhythmic tremor of the limbs which subsides on active movement. The speech may become indistinct.

TREATMENT. The treatment of parkinsonism is mainly symptomatic, with belladonna alkaloids or with synthetic drugs having belladonna-like effects. Diphenhydramine (Benadryl) may be used as adjunctive medication and amphetamines or imipramine are added to alleviate depression.

L-DOPA. Norepinephrine, dopamine, 5-hydroxytryptamine, acetylcholine and $\gamma$-aminobutyric acid are chemical substances thought to be concerned with neurotransmission. Norepinephrine and 5-hydroxytryptamine are found particularly in the hypothalamus, but dopamine is present in largest amounts in parts of the basal ganglia. In parkinsonism the concentration of dopamine is significantly reduced. Dopamine was given by mouth in an attempt to increase its concentration in the brain but it was found that it does not reach the central nervous system. It has been found that L-dopa which is metabolized to dopamine produces partial improvement in all patients with parkinsonism and dramatic improvement in some (Annotation, 1969).

Surgical treatment consists of making a destructive lesion in the globus pallidus or anterior thalamus. It has been employed in unilateral involvement in patients under age 60 in whom there is no evidence of cerebral atherosclerosis.

## Hepatolenticular Degeneration

Hepatolenticular degeneration is characterized by cavitation in the lenticular nuclei, cirrhosis of the liver, and incoordination and tremors of the extremities associated with a ring of greenish brown or golden brown discoloration of the periphery of the cornea (Kayser-Fleischer ring). The disease results from an inborn error of metabolism, characterized by a deficiency in the blood of the copper-binding protein, ceruloplasmin, and by amino-aciduria. Deposition of copper occurs in the brain, liver and cornea.

## FITS AND FAINTS IN THE DENTAL OFFICE

Consciousness may be clouded or lost as the result of a fit which is neurologic in origin or of a faint which is cardiovascular in origin. In addition there are other causes such a hypoglycemia and internal hemorrhage.

### Fit

The occurrence of jerky movements and not merely stiffness suggests that the attack is a fit or epileptiform attack. Incontinence of urine, tongue biting, injury in the attack and scars on the tongue also point towards a diagnosis of epilepsy (see p. 175).

### Faint

In all the conditions of cardiovascular origin in which consciousness is lost, the mechanism is a period of cardiac asystole or arrhythmia or of low blood pressure (50 mms. Hg.). Tonic rigidity of the muscles may occur but there are no real clonic movements.

There are two main groups of faints:

1. Where there is evidence of heart disease, such as heart block and aortic incompetence. Patients with these forms of heart disease may faint after moderate exertion.
2. Where there is no evidence of heart disease, such as simple fainting or syncope, postural syncope, carotid sinus syncope and cough syncope.

## SYNCOPE

Syncope may occur as a result of emotional strain or a hot atmosphere. It is characterized by a gradual onset, preceded by pallor, a cold sweat and a fast weak pulse.

## POSTURAL SYNCOPE

Postural syncope occurs in susceptible patients who lose consciousness on changing from a lying down position to a vertical position. It may be induced by ganglion blocking agents and phenothiazines.

## CAROTID SINUS SYNCOPE

Certain individuals have increased sensitivity of the carotid sinus and syncopal attacks may occur when the patient is wearing a tight collar and suddenly turns his head to one side, thus stimulating the carotid sinus and producing vagal slowing of the heart.

## COUGH SYNCOPE

Syncope may follow a bout of coughing in some plethoric, emphysematous middle-aged males. This condition results from a rise in the intrathoracic pressure which impedes venous return. The latter causes a decrease of cardiac output and a fall of blood pressure sufficient to cause cerebral anoxia.

### Other Kinds of Attack

Two common types of attack are:

## HYPOGLYCEMIA

The patient may have taken his normal dose of insulin and not followed it soon enough by a meal. Convulsive seizures may occur that are identical with those in idiopathic epilepsy.

## INTERNAL HEMORRHAGE FROM A PEPTIC ULCER

The patient may have a history of dyspepsia. There is increasing pallor, rising pulse rate and falling blood pressure associated with dyspnea and restlessness.

## GENERAL REFERENCES

Annotation: Dopa in Parkinson's disease. Lancet, *i.*, 87[1], 1969.
Balla, J. I. and Walton, J. N.: Periodic migrainous neuralgia. Brit. Med. J., *1*, 219, 1964.
Beaver, D. L., Moses, H. L., and Ganote, C. E.: Electron microscopy of the trigeminal ganglion. Arch. Path., *79*, 557, 1965.
Birch, A. C.: 'Fits, faints and unconsciousness,' in *Emergencies in Medical Practice* (Ed. C. A. Birch), 8th ed., Edinburgh, Livingstone, 1967, pp. 244–248.
Brodal, A.: *The Cranial Nerves. Anatomy and Anatomico-Clinical Correlations,* 2nd ed. Oxford, Blackwell Scientific Publications, 1957.
Gardner, J. S. and Dohn, D. F.: Trigeminal neuralgia-hemifacial spasm. Paget's disease—significance of the association. Brain, *89*, 555, 1966.
Kennett, S. and Cohen, L.: Paroxysmal trigeminal neuralgia. A review of 36 cases. Oral Surg., *25*, 2, 1968.
Lascelles, R. G.: Atypical facial pain and depression. Brit. J. Psychiat., *112*, 651, 1966.
Laskin, D. M.: Etiology of the pain-dysfunction syndrome. JADA, *79*, 147, 1969.
Matthews, W. B.: *Practical Neurology*, Oxford, Blackwell Scientific Publications, 1963.
Plum, F.: 'Headache' in *Cecil-Loeb Textbook of Medicine* (Eds. P. B. Beeson and W. McDermott), 13th ed., Philadelphia, Saunders, 1971, pp. 154–160.

## SUGGESTED READING

Symposium on Facial Pain Issue. Headache, *9*, 1, April 1969.

## Chapter 14

# THE MEDICAL ASPECTS OF HEAD INJURIES

After a mild head injury, the patient may be momentarily confused and then carry on his activities automatically and attract little attention from onlookers. When he recovers from this automatic state, he may be unable to recall any of his activities since the injury (amnesia).

It is convenient to classify amnesia into two types: *Retrograde amnesia* is lack of memory for events leading up to the accident. *Anterograde amnesia* is lack of memory for events following the accident. The greater the degree of anterograde amnesia, the more severe the structural damage to the brain tissue is likely to be.

Occasionally a mild injury may produce no immediate symptoms but several hours later there may be confusion, dizziness, vomiting and brady-cardia. The condition usually resolves after a few hours but may persist for several days.

In mild head injury the prognosis is excellent but extradural hemorrhage is almost invariably fatal unless it is recognized promptly and dealt with by a neurosurgeon (see p. 177).

## CEREBRAL STATE OF THE PATIENT FOLLOWING A HEAD INJURY

This may be classified in the following manner:
1. *Conscious*
    a. Clear, in which case the patient is rational
    b. Confused, in which case the patient is disoriented in time and place
2. *Unconscious*
    a. Semi-comatose
    b. Comatose

13

## The Patient Is Conscious

*Confusion* may be defined as a clouding of consciousness. When moderate confusion exists, the patient is disoriented but can accurately answer simple questions regarding his name, age and address. Severe confusion occurs when the patient is inaccessible for the greater part of the time but will occasionally respond to repeated commands.

## The Patient Is Unconscious

### SEMI-COMA

In this condition the patient is completely uncooperative but will respond to painful stimuli such as pressure over the supraorbital nerve. The corneal and swallowing reflexes are still present but frequently there is retention of urine with overflow.

### COMA

In this state, there is no response to pain and in severe cases, all the reflexes are absent. Reflex emptying of the bladder occurs following distention of this organ. If there is severe brain damage, death may ensue. In those patients who survive, return of consciousness may occur within minutes or hours or may be delayed for days. As the patient recovers, he passes through a stage of cerebral irritation in which he lies curled up on his side and avoids the light because of photophobia. He may violently resist examination or nursing attention.

## OTHER CAUSES OF UNCONSCIOUSNESS BESIDES HEAD INJURY

These include alcohol, epilepsy, diabetic or insulin coma, uremia, overdosage with barbiturates and cerebrovascular accidents (CVA).

The fixed, dilated pupil of Hutchinson is a reliable sign of raised intracranial pressure. Following a rise of intracranial pressure, the pupil on the affected side dilates but still reacts to light. Unless the intracranial pressure is relieved, the pupil dilates further and no longer reacts to light either directly or consensually. Finally, the opposite pupil becomes widely dilated and fixed and death is imminent.

## MANAGEMENT OF HEAD INJURIES

### Pulse

A continuous half-hourly record of the pulse should be instituted in order to recognize an increase of intracranial pressure. As the pressure rises, the pulse rate at first increases but later it decreases. If the patient is unconscious and the pulse rate is below 60 per minute, increased intracranial pressure is present. A possible diagnosis to consider is extradural hemorrhage.

## Blood Pressure

Half-hourly blood pressure readings should be taken. If the patient becomes more drowsy and the pulse rate full and bounding, the systolic blood pressure slowly increases and continues to rise as the pulse rate falls. The diastolic pressure does not rise proportionately and may remain dangerously low. In the terminal stages, the pulse becomes more rapid and feeble, the blood pressure falls suddenly and death ensues.

## Temperature

This may be slightly raised (99°–100° F). Should a further rise of temperature occur after a day or so, this may indicate further hemorrhage or the onset of meningeal infection.

## Respiration

Increasing intracranial pressure causes ischemia of the respiratory center in the medulla and an alteration of the normal respiratory rhythm occurs. Marked deviation from the normal rhythm carries a poor prognosis as does stertor, which is essentially due to a loss of muscle tone allowing the jaw and tongue to fall backwards and thus obstruct the airway. In the terminal stages, Cheyne-Stokes respiration occurs.

# TREATMENT OF A HEAD INJURY NOT REQUIRING NEUROSURGERY

The immediate treatment will be primarily concerned with the maintenance of the airway, the arrest of any severe hemorrhage, treatment of primary shock and the prevention of infection. The nasopharynx should be cleared of mucus and blood clots by means of a suction apparatus. If the foot of the bed is raised and the patient is nursed on his side, secretions pool in the nasopharynx and may be removed. The patient should be turned every four hours in order to drain the dependent lung and to minimize the risk of bed sores. In the presence of severe respiratory obstruction, a tracheostomy is indicated.

If consciousness has not been regained after 12 hours, the patient should be fed intravenously. Feeding by nasal tube can be started within 48 hours. Oral feeding should commence as soon as possible.

## Sedation

Restlessness is often due to a full bladder and a patient will usually settle down when this cause of irritation has been relieved. Chlorpromazine (25 mg.) can be given at intervals of two hours as needed. Paraldehyde (6 ml.) can be given by rectum or deeply into the gluteal muscle. If there is pain, 32 mg. codeine can be given but not morphine which depresses respiration and deepens coma.

## Convalescence

The patient is allowed up when he has been free from headache for about four days. Initially, the patient should be out of bed for short periods only and if there is a recurrence of the headaches or if he complains of nausea or dizziness, he should be put back to bed again.

### Treatment of Associated Maxillo-Facial Injuries

In the presence of a head injury, it is wiser to defer treatment of the maxillo-facial injury for 24 or 48 hours before administering an anesthetic.

### Lumbar Puncture

This is potentially dangerous in the presence of raised intracranial pressure as withdrawal of cerebrospinal fluid carries with it the potential risk of forcing the cerebellar tonsils into the foramen magnum with sudden death.

### Associated Injuries

It must be remembered that the patient may have other injuries in addition to the head injury. A careful examination is necessary to exclude the possibility of chest injuries, ruptured abdominal viscera and fractures of extremities.

## THE LATE COMPLICATIONS OF HEAD INJURY

Symptoms such as headache, dizziness, poor concentration, memory defects and personality changes principally manifested by emotional instability may be encountered. Some cranial nerve injuries arising as a result of the head injury may persist.

Post-traumatic epilepsy due to the formation of scar tissue in the brain or meninges may be a late complication of head injuries, the average time of incidence for which is approximately one year following injury.

## GENERAL REFERENCES

Rowe, N. L. and Killey, H. C.: *Fractures of the Facial Skeleton*, 2nd ed., Baltimore, Williams & Wilkins, 1968, pp. 634–644.
Simpson, J. A.: 'Neurological emergencies,' in *Emergencies in Medical Practice* (Ed. C. A. Birch), 8th ed., Edinburgh, Livingstone, 1967, pp, 249–285.

## SUGGESTED READING

Jackson, F. E.: *The Treatment of Head Injuries*, Ciba Foundation, 1967.

Chapter 15

# SOME DRUGS USED IN THERAPY

## ANTIBIOTICS

An antibiotic is a chemical substance produced either by microorganisms or by synthetic methods which is capable of inhibiting the growth of or destroying other microorganisms.

It is convenient to divide antibiotics into two groups, bacteriostatic and bactericidal agents. A *bacteriostatic* drug is one which prevents the growth of organisms in the host thereby allowing the body's natural defense mechanisms to overcome the infection. A *bactericidal* drug actively kills bacteria which are eliminated with the aid of the body's defenses. It is possible for an antibiotic to be bacteriostatic in low concentrations and bactericidal in high concentrations as in the case of penicillin.

Bactericidal drugs are to be preferred when possible as they are effective more rapidly, may be synergistic when used in combination against bacteria which are difficult to eliminate, and are less likely to leave resistant organisms. Antagonism between chemotherapeutic agents is of little clinical importance.

*Primarily bactericidal antibiotics* include penicillin, streptomycin, bacitracin, neomycin and erythromycin (high concentration).

*Primarily bacteriostatic antibiotics* are the tetracyclines, erythromycin (low concentration), chloramphenicol and sulfonamides.

## MODE OF ACTION OF ANTIBACTERIAL DRUGS

The penicillins and cephalosporins interfere with bacterial cell wall synthesis. Protein manufacture by the bacterial cell is interfered with by

187

the tetracyclines, chloramphenicol, erythromycin, lincomycin and strepto-mycin. Streptomycin, kanamycin and neomycin also cause the organism to manufacture abnormal proteins.

Penicillin and the erythromycin group are most useful against gram-positive microorganisms and the streptomycin group against the gram-negative organisms and tubercle bacillus. Broad-spectrum antibiotics such as tetracyclines and chloramphenicol are effective in both gram-positive and gram-negative infections and also against the rickettsia.

## SEMISYNTHETIC PENICILLINS

The penicillin-producing mold is allowed to produce the active penicillin nucleus (6-aminopenicillanic acid), and different side chains are attached to the nucleus by the chemist and give rise to the group of semisynthetic penicillins. Phenoxymethyl penicillin and methicillin are resistant to gastric acid and may be given by mouth in less severe infections. Methi-cillin, oxacillin, nafcillin and cloxacillin are not destroyed by staphylococcal penicillinase and may be employed in infections due to these organisms. Ampicillin is effective in gram-positive and gram-negative infections. Patients who are sensitive to penicillin G will also react to the semisyn-thetic penicillins.

## ERYTHROMYCIN

Erythromycin is used as an alternative to penicillin in penicillin-sensitive individuals.

## LINCOMYCIN

Lincomycin is currently employed in bone infections caused by penicilli-nase-producing strains of staphylococci or penicillin-resistant pathogenic streptococci.

## CEPHALOSPORINS

These are a number of antibiotics related to penicillin. They are active against gram-positive and most gram-negative organisms and are used in penicillin-sensitive individuals. This, however, is not without danger as some of these patients may also have allergic reactions to the cephalosporins. Cephalothin sodium (Keflin) is a member of this group.

## TETRACYCLINES

The members of this group resemble each other in their antibacterial activity. For this reason when a tetracycline is indicated any member of the group may be prescribed. These drugs cause discoloration of the de-veloping teeth. Demeclocycline has the advantage that it can be given twice a day instead of four times as with the other tetracyclines. The drug may induce an exaggerated sunburn reaction in certain sensitive individuals.

## CHLORAMPHENICOL

Chloramphenicol may cause thrombocytopenic purpura, aplastic anemia and agranulocytosis.

## MYCOSTATIN

When used in the treatment of oral candidiasis, mycostatin tablets should be sucked as they exert a local action only.

## ANTIBIOTIC OINTMENTS

Neomycin, bacitracin, polymyxin B, tyrothricin, mycostatin and aureomycin ointments are used for the local treatment of infections. In the treatment of angular cheilitis due to bacteria, three-percent aureomycin ointment is useful and is less likely to produce sensitization than other antibiotics.

### Sulfonamides

These drugs have no place in the treatment of dental infections; they are used in gastrointestinal and urinary infections. They are also indicated in the prevention of meningeal infection after a fracture of the cribriform plate of the ethmoid occurring in severe facial injuries. As a result of the frac-

### Table 1. Antibiotic Dosages

| Antibiotic | Usual Adult Dose |
| --- | --- |
| Penicillin G | 250,000 to 1,000,000 units or more intramuscularly q 3 hours |
| Penicillin G procaine (Duracillin A. S., Wycillin) | 300,000 to 1,200,000 units intramuscularly once a day |
| Penicillin G benzathine (Bicillin) | 600,000 units intramuscularly every 2–3 weeks (rheumatic fever prophylaxis) |
| Phenoxymethyl penicillin (Pen·Vee Oral, V-Cillin) | 250–500 mg. q.i.d. orally |
| Cloxacillin sodium monohydrate (Tegopen) | 0.5–1.0 gm. q 4–6 hours orally |
| Nafcillin sodium (Unipen) | 0.5–1.0 gm. q.i.d. orally, intramuscularly or intravenously |
| Ampicillin (Polycillin, Totacillin) | 250–500 mg. q.i.d. orally, intramuscularly or intravenously |
| Cephalothin sodium (Keflin) | 0.5–1.0 gm. q.i.d. intramuscularly or intravenously |
| Erythromycin (Ilotycin, Erythrocin) | 250 mg. q.i.d. orally |
| Lincomycin hydrochloride monohydrate (Lincocin) | 500 mg. q.i.d. orally or 600 mg. b.i.d. intramuscularly or intravenously |
| Tetracycline (Achromycin, Tetracyn) | 250 mg. q.i.d. orally |
| Chlortetracycline hydrochloride (Aureomycin) | 250 mg. q.i.d. orally |
| Oxytetracycline (Terramycin) | 250 mg. q.i.d. orally |
| Demeclocycline hydrochloride (Declomycin) | 300 mg. b.i.d. orally |
| Mycostatin tablets | 1 tablet (500,000 units) to be sucked q.i.d. |

ture organisms can pass with ease from the nose into the cranial cavity. The drug of choice is sulfadiazine—4 gm. initially by mouth, then 1 gm. every 4 hours for maintenance. The risk of crystal formation in the urine can be minimized by ensuring that the patient has a daily fluid intake of at least two liters (four pints).

See p. 18 for drug allergy and for dermatologic allergy.

## ANALGESIC AGENTS

Analgesic agents include non-narcotic and narcotic analgesics. The salicylates and para-aminophenol derivatives in addition to their analgesic activity will lower a raised temperature (antipyretic analgesics).

### Table 2.   Analgesic Agents

| Analgesic | Usual Adult Dose |
| --- | --- |
| Acetylsalicylic acid (Aspirin) | 0.3–1.0 gm. q 4 hours orally |
| Acetaminophen (Tempra, Tylenol) | 0.3–0.6 gm. q 4 hours orally |
| Propoxyphene (Darvon) | 65 mg. t.i.d. or q.i.d. orally |
| Codeine sulfate or phosphate | 30–60 mg. q 4 hours orally |
| Meperidine hydrochloride (Demerol hydrochloride) | 50–100 mg. q 4 hours orally or intramuscularly |
| Pentazocine hydrochloride (Talwin hydrochloride) | 30 mg. q 4 hours subcutaneously or intramuscularly |
| Morphine sulfate | 5–15 mg. q 4 hours subcutaneously |

### Narcotic Antagonists

Nalorphine hydrochloride (Nalline hydrochloride)—5–10 mg. intravenously—and levallorphan tartrate (Lorfan)—1–2 mg. intravenously—are used as antidotes in overdosage with any narcotic analgesic.

## ANTIHISTAMINES

The main actions of histamine are to cause contraction of smooth muscle, dilatation of capillaries with leakage of plasma, and secretion of hydrochloric acid. The antihistamines oppose all the actions of histamine with the exception of the secretion of hydrochloric acid in the stomach.

The antihistamines are used in the treatment of urticaria, hayfever and some allergic skin diseases. For acute anaphylactic type reactions they are not as effective as epinephrine.

SIDE EFFECTS. Some degree of drowsiness is almost invariable and it may be severe. Inability to concentrate, dizziness and disturbances of coordination and dryness of the mouth are other common side effects.

A large number of antihistamines are available but the three drugs listed in Table 3 are adequate for most purposes.

### Table 3.  Antihistamines

| Drug | By Intramuscular Injection | Usual Adult Dose (Oral) |
|---|---|---|
| Chlorpheniramine maleate (Chlor-Trimeton) | 10 mg. | 4 mg. t.i.d. or q.i.d. |
| Diphenhydramine hydrochloride (Benadryl) | 10–50 mg. | 50 mg. t.i.d. or q.i.d. |
| Promethazine hydrochloride (Phenergan) | 12.5–25 mg. | 25 mg. at bedtime |

## SEDATIVES AND HYPNOTICS

Included in this group are both the barbiturate and nonbarbiturate sedatives and hypnotics.  Some of the barbiturates listed in Table 4 as hypnotics may be used as sedatives by giving half the dose.

### Table 4.  Sedatives and Hypnotics

| Drug | Usual Adult Dose |
|---|---|
| BARBITURATES | |
| Phenobarbital | 30 to 60 mg., 1 to 4 times a day orally as a sedative, 100–200 mg. as a hypnotic |
| Amobarbital (Amytal) | 100–200 mg. orally as a hypnotic |
| Pentobarbital (Nembutal) | 100–200 mg. orally as a hypnotic |
| Secobarbital (Seconal) | 100–200 mg. orally as a hypnotic |
| NONBARBITURATES | |
| Chloral hydrate | 0.5–2.0 gm. orally as a hypnotic |
| Paraldehyde | 4–8 ml. intramuscularly as a sedative |
| Glutethimide (Doriden) | 500 mg.–1 gm. orally as a hypnotic |

## TRANQUILIZERS

Tranquilizers are divided into two groups, major and minor.  Major tranquilizers include the phenothiazine derivatives such as chlorpromazine (Thorazine) and promazine hydrochloride (Sparine) and are used in the treatment of psychoses.  These drugs produce dry mouth and in some cases symptoms of Parkinsonism.  Bizarre involuntary movements of the facial muscles may occur in some patients taking these drugs.  Among the minor tranquilizers are meprobamate (Equanil, Miltown), chlordiazepoxide hydrochloride (Librium) and diazepam (Valium) which are used in the treatment of anxiety states.

### Table 5.  Tranquilizers

| Drug | |
|---|---|
| Chlorpromazine (Thorazine) | 10–25 mg. t.i.d. orally |
| Promazine hydrochloride (Sparine) | 25–50 mg. q.i.d. orally |
| Meprobamate (Equanil, Miltown) | 400 mg. t.i.d. or q.i.d. orally |
| Chlordiazepoxide hydrochloride (Librium) | 5–10 mg. t.i.d. or q.i.d. orally |
| Diazepam (Valium) | 2–10 mg. b.i.d. or t.i.d. orally |

## MONOAMINE OXIDASE INHIBITORS

These drugs were used in the treatment of depression but are now largely replaced by the tricyclic compounds such as imipramine. The monoamine oxidase inhibitors potentiate the effects of narcotics such as morphine and meperidine. It is necessary to stop administration of these drugs at least two weeks before surgery.

## GLUCOCORTICOIDS

Glucocorticoids may be used locally or systemically. They are employed for physiologic replacement in adrenal insufficiency (Addison's disease) and following adrenalectomy together with a mineralocorticoid. In addition they suppress certain pathologic states and are used in the collagen diseases, hypersensitivity reactions (asthma, serum sickness), hemolytic anemia, drug reactions, agranulocytosis, acute leukemia, some eye diseases, ulcerative colitis, exfoliative dermatitis and pemphigus.

Glucocorticoids are contraindicated in patients with a history of peptic ulceration as they increase gastric acid secretion and may reactivate an ulcer which may bleed or perforate without warning. In patients with healed tuberculosis, dissemination of the disease may occur because of the suppression of the inflammatory response and interference with the immune mechanism.

Equivalent dosages of glucocorticoids are: cortisone, 25 mg.; hydrocortisone, 20 mg.; prednisone, 5 mg.; prednisolone, 5 mg.; triamcinoline, 4 mg.; paramethasone, 2 mg.; and dexamethasone, 0.75 mg.

It should be noted that after about six weeks of treatment with glucocorticoids, suppression of the patient's own adrenals occurs. Abrupt withdrawal produces a hypoadrenal state and it is therefore necessary to decrease the dose of the drug gradually when therapy is discontinued. Usually adrenal function is restored within a few weeks, but occasionally relative adrenal insufficiency may persist for as long as one year.

Prolonged dosage with glucocorticoids may lead to symptoms of Cushing's syndrome (see p. 136).

## ORAL SURGERY IN PATIENTS WITH ADRENAL INSUFFICIENCY

Each day the human adrenal cortex secretes about 25 mg. of cortisol. Under the stress of a general anesthetic, a surgical procedure or an infection the output of cortisol may rise to 200 to 300 mg. If the patient is currently taking a glucocorticoid or ACTH or has adrenal suppression because of a course of these drugs during the previous two years a fatal adrenal crisis may be precipitated from failure of the patient's adrenals to respond to the body's demand for extra cortisol. To prevent this, prophylactic steroid cover should be given before an oral surgical procedure on a patient with adrenal insufficiency is undertaken. The patient's physician should be consulted and it may be necessary to admit the patient to the hospital.

A suitable regimen is to administer 100 mg. cortisone acetate intramuscularly the evening before the oral surgery and three interspaced 100 mg. doses of cortisone acetate intramuscularly on the day of the operation. The dose can then be reduced gradually each day until the maintenance dosage level is reached, or tapered off completely within seven to ten days in a patient who has resumed steroid therapy to cover the period of operation.

## ANTICOAGULANT DRUGS

Anticoagulant drugs are used in the treatment of recurrent thrombotic disease, postoperative thrombophlebitis, pulmonary embolism and coronary thrombosis. The drugs in common use are derivatives of coumarin and indandione and they act by interfering with the synthesis of prothrombin in the liver probably by competition with vitamin K. Hematuria, rectal bleeding and epistaxis may occur in patients receiving anticoagulant drugs. If bleeding appears, the intravenous administration of vitamin K (Mephyton) in a dose of 10 to 50 mg. will reverse the hypoprothrombinemia in three to six hours.

## TOOTH EXTRACTION IN PATIENTS RECEIVING ANTICOAGULANT DRUGS

The patient's physician should always be consulted. It is dangerous to terminate the anticoagulant drugs abruptly as in some patients a hypercoagulable state ('rebound thrombosis') occurs which may be fatal. Extraction of a tooth has been performed without lowering the dose of anticoagulant. The socket is sutured, pressure is applied and the patient is advised not to rinse his mouth for 24 hours. Some authorities prefer to reduce the anticoagulant drug to bring the prothrombin time (normal, 12–15 seconds) to about $1\frac{1}{2}$ times normal and then extract the tooth.

## ADMINISTRATION OF DRUGS TO CHILDREN

In prescribing drugs for children the dosage can be obtained by Young's rule which is:

$$\text{Child dose} = \frac{\text{age} \times \text{adult dose}}{\text{age} + 12}$$

A second formula is Clark's rule:

$$\text{Child dose} = \frac{\text{Weight of child in lbs.} \times \text{adult dose}}{150}$$

The dose for aspirin (acetylsalicylic acid) is 1 gr. (0.06 gm.) per year of age up to five years and may be repeated as often as every four hours if necessary.

Phenobarbital is widely used as a sedative. Elixir of phenobarbital has $\frac{1}{4}$ gr. (15 mg.) per teaspoon. Infants take $\frac{1}{8}$ to $\frac{1}{4}$ gr. (8 to 15 mg.) well, and it is rarely necessary to use dosages greater than $\frac{1}{2}$ gr. (30 mg.) on children.

The usual dosages for analgesia of codeine, morphine, meperidine hydrochloride (Demerol) and paregoric are: codeine, 3 mg. per kg. per day, orally or subcutaneously; morphine, 0.1 to 0.2 mg. per kg. per dose, subcutaneously; paregoric (0.4 mg. morphine per ml.), 0.25 to 0.5 ml. per kg. per dose, orally; meperidine (Demerol), 6 mg. per kg. per day, orally or subcutaneously.

## GENERAL REFERENCES

*Accepted Dental Therapeutics*, 33rd ed., Chicago, American Dental Association, 1970.

*AMA Drug Evaluations*, Chicago, American Medical Association, 1971.

Cutting, W. C.: *Handbook of Pharmacology*, 3rd ed., New York, Appleton-Century-Crofts, 1969.

Slobody, L. B. and Wasserman, E.: *Survey of Clinical Pediatrics*, 5th ed., New York, McGraw-Hill, 1968, pp. 76–99.

## SUGGESTED READING

Kay, L. W.: *Drugs in Dentistry*. Bristol, Wright, 1969.

# INDEX

195